INTRODUCTION

To the Self-Instructional Workbook

Paramedic Care: Principles & Practice

Welcome to the self-instructional workbook for *Paramedic Care: Principles & Practice*. This workbook is designed to help guide you through an educational program for initial or refresher training that follows the guidelines of the 1998 U.S. Department of Transportation EMT-Paramedic National Standard Curriculum. The workbook is designed to be used either in conjunction with your instructor or as a self-study guide you use on your own.

This workbook features many different ways to help you learn the material necessary to become a paramedic, including those listed below.

FEATURES

Review of Chapter Objectives

Each chapter of *Paramedic Care: Principles & Practice* begins with objectives that identify the important information and principles addressed in the chapter reading. To help you identify and learn this material, each workbook chapter reviews the important content elements addressed by these objectives as presented in the text.

Case Study Review

Each chapter of *Paramedic Care: Principles & Practice* includes a case study, introducing and highlighting important principles presented in the chapter. The workbook reviews these case studies and points out much of the essential information and many of the applied principles they describe.

Content Self-Evaluation

Each chapter of *Paramedic Care: Principles & Practice* presents an extensive narrative explanation of the principles of paramedic practice. The workbook chapter (or chapter section) contains between 10 and 50 multiple-choice questions to test your reading comprehension of the textbook material and to give you experience taking typical emergency medical service examinations.

Special Projects

The workbook contains several projects that are special learning experiences designed to help you remember the information and principles necessary to perform as a paramedic. Special projects include crossword puzzles, prehospital care reports completion, personal benchmarking activities, and a variety of other exercises.

Prehospital Care Reports

The workbook provides you with narrative information regarding simulated calls and then asks you to record that information on prehospital care report forms. These exercises help you refine your ability to identify important medical information and record it on the prehospital care reports as you would in real life situations.

Personal Benchmarking

The workbook provides several exercises that direct you to evaluate elements of the patient assessment process on yourself. These exercises help you develop your assessment skills and to use normal findings as benchmarks for reference when you begin your career as a paramedic.

Chapter Sections

Several chapters in *Paramedic Care: Principles & Practice* are long and contain a great deal of subject matter. To help you grasp this material more efficiently, the workbook breaks these chapters into sections with their own objectives, content review, and special projects.

Content Review

The workbook provides a comprehensive review of the material presented in this volume of *Paramedic Care: Principles & Practice*. After the last text chapter has been covered, the workbook presents an extensive content self-evaluation component that helps you recall and build upon the knowledge you have gained by reading the text, attending class, and completing the earlier workbook chapters.

National Registry Practical Evaluation Forms

Supplemental materials found at the back of the workbook include the National Registry Practical Evaluation Forms. These or similar forms will be used to test your practical skills throughout your training and, usually, for state certification exams. By reviewing them, you have a clearer picture of what is expected of you during your practical exam and a better understanding of the type of evaluation tool that is used to measure your performance.

Patient Scenario Flash Cards

At the end of this workbook are scenario flash cards, which are designed to help you practice the processes of investigating both the chief complaint and the past medical history. Each card contains the dispatch information and results of the scene survey and then prompts you to inquire into either the patient's major symptoms or his or her past medical history.

ACKNOWLEDGMENTS

Reviewers
The reviewers listed below provided many excellent suggestions for improving this workbook. Their assistance is greatly appreciated.

Blaine Griffiths, BSAS, RN, NREMT-P
Youngstown State University

David M. Habben, NREMT-P
EMS Consultant
Boise, Idaho

Matthew R. Streger, MPA, NREMT-P
Paramedic
Greenville County Emergency Medical Services
Greenville, South Carolina

BRADY

PARAMEDIC CARE: PRINCIPLES & PRACTICE

PATIENT ASSESSMENT

Workbook

Robert S. Porter

BRYAN E. BLEDSOE, D.O., F.A.C.E.P., F.A.A.E.M., F.A.E.P., EMT-P
Emergency Department Staff Physician
Baylor Medical Center—Ellis County
Waxahachie, Texas
and
Clinical Associate Professor of Emergency Medicine
University of North Texas Health Sciences Center
Fort Worth, Texas

ROBERT S. PORTER, M.A., NREMT-P
Senior Advanced Life Support Educator
Madison County Emergency Medical Services
Canastota, New York
and
Flight Paramedic
AirOne, Onondaga County Sheriff's Department
Syracuse, New York

RICHARD A. CHERRY, M.S., NREMT-P
Clinical Assistant Professor of Emergency Medicine
Director of Paramedic Training
SUNY Upstate Medical University
Syracuse, New York

Brady
Prentice Hall Health
Upper Saddle River, NJ 07458

Dedication

*To Kris and Sailing: Pleasant distractions from writing about
and practicing prehospital emergency medicine.*

PUBLISHER: *Julie Alexander*
ACQUISITIONS EDITOR: *Laura Edwards*
MANAGING DEVELOPMENT EDITOR: *Lois Berlowitz*
DEVELOPMENT EDITOR: *Dan Zinkus*
MARKETING MANAGER: *Tiffany Price*
DIRECTOR OF MANUFACTURING & PRODUCTION:
   Bruce Johnson
SENIOR PRODUCTION MANAGER: *Ilene Sanford*
MANAGING PRODUCTION EDITOR: *Patrick Walsh*
PRODUCTION EDITOR: *Larry Hayden*
PRODUCTION SUPERVISION: *Navta Associates, Inc.*
PRINTER/BINDER: *Banta Harrisonburg*

 © 2000 by Prentice-Hall, Inc.
Upper Saddle River, New Jersey 07458

Printed in the United States of America
10 9 8 7 6 5 4 3

ISBN 0-13-021632-1

Prentice-Hall International (UK) Limited, *London*
Prentice-Hall of Australia Pty. Limited, *Sydney*
Prentice-Hall Canada Inc., *Toronto*
Prentice-Hall Hispanoamericana, S.A., *Mexico*
Prentice-Hall of India Private Limited, *New Delhi*
Prentice-Hall of Japan, Inc., *Tokyo*
Prentice-Hall (Singapore) Pte Ltd
Editora Prentice-Hall do Brasil, Ltda., *Rio de Janeiro*

NOTICE ON CARE PROCEDURES

It is the intent of the authors and publisher that this workbook be used as part of a formal EMT-Paramedic program taught by qualified instructors and supervised by a licensed physician. The procedures described in this workbook are based upon consultation with EMT and medical authorities. The authors and publisher have taken care to make certain that these procedures reflect currently accepted clinical practice; however, they cannot be considered absolute recommendations.

The material in this workbook contains the most current information available at the time of publication. However, federal, state, and local guidelines concerning clinical practices, including, without limitation, those governing infection control and universal precautions, change rapidly. The reader should note, therefore, that the new regulations may require changes in some procedures.

It is the responsibility of the reader to familiarize himself or herself with the policies and procedures set by federal, state, and local agencies as well as the institution or agency where the reader is employed. The authors and the publisher of this workbook disclaim any liability, loss, or risk resulting directly or indirectly from the suggested procedures and theory, from any undetected errors, or from the reader's misunderstanding of the text. It is the reader's responsibility to stay informed of any new changes or recommendations made by any federal, state, and local agency as well as by his or her employing institution or agency.

CONTENTS

Self-Instructional Workbook

Paramedic Care: Principles & Practice

PATIENT ASSESSMENT

How to Use
The Self-Instructional Workbook
Paramedic Care: Principles & Practice

The self-instructional workbook accompanying *Paramedic Care: Principles & Practice* may be used as directed by your instructor or independently by you during your course of instruction. The recommendations listed below are intended to guide you in using the workbook independently.

- Examine your course schedule and identify the appropriate text chapter or other assigned reading.

- Read the assigned chapter in *Paramedic Care: Principles & Practice* carefully. Do this in a relaxed environment, free of distractions, and give yourself adequate time to read and digest the material. The information presented in *Paramedic Care: Principles & Practice* is often technically complex and demanding, but it is very important that you comprehend it. Be sure that you read the chapter carefully enough to understand and remember what you have read.

- Carefully read the Review of Chapter Objectives at the beginning of each workbook chapter (or section). This material includes both the objectives listed in *Paramedic Care: Principles & Practice* and narrative descriptions of their content. If you do not understand or remember what is discussed from your reading, refer to the referenced pages and reread them carefully. If you still do not feel comfortable with your understanding of any objective, consider asking your instructor about it.

- Reread the case study in *Paramedic Care: Principles & Practice,* and then read the Case Study Review in the workbook. Note the important points regarding assessment and care that the Case Study Review highlights, and be sure that you understand and agree with the analysis of the call. If you have any questions or concerns, ask your instructor to clarify the information.

- Take the Content Self-Evaluation at the end of each workbook chapter (or section), answering each question carefully. Do this in a quiet environment, free from distractions, and allow yourself adequate time to complete the exercise. Correct your self-evaluation by consulting the answers at the back of the workbook, and determine the percentage you have answered correctly (the number you got right divided by the total number of questions). If you have answered most of the questions correctly (85 to 90 percent), review those that you missed by rereading the material on the pages listed in the answer key and be sure you understand which answer is correct and why. If you have more than a few questions wrong (less than 85 percent correct), look for incorrect answers that are grouped together. This suggests that you did not understand a particular topic in the reading. Reread the text dealing with that topic carefully, and then retest yourself on the questions you got wrong. If incorrect answers are spread throughout the chapter content, reread the chapter and re-take the Content Self-Evaluation to assure that you understand the material. If you don't understand why your answer to a question is incorrect after reviewing the text, consult with your instructor.

- In a similar fashion, complete the exercises in the Special Projects section of the workbook chapters (or sections). These exercises are specifically designed to help you learn and remember the essential principles and information presented in *Paramedic Care: Principles & Practice*.

- When you have completed this volume of *Paramedic Care: Principles & Practice* and its accompanying workbook, prepare for a course test by reviewing both the text in its entirety and your class notes. Then take the Content Review examination in the workbook and complete the associated Special Projects. Again, review your score and any questions you have answered incorrectly by referring to the text and rereading the page or pages where the material is presented. If you note groupings of wrong answers, review the entire range of pages or the full chapter they represent.

If, during your completion of the workbook exercises, you have any questions that either the text-book or workbook doesn't answer, write them down and ask your instructor about them. Prehospital emergency medicine is a complex and complicated subject, and answers are not always black-and-white. It is also common for different EMS systems to use differing methods of care. The questions you bring up in class, and your instructor's answers to them, will help you expand and complete your knowledge of prehospital emergency medical care.

The authors and Brady Publishing continuously seek to assure the creation of the best materials to support your educational experience. We are interested in your comments. If, during your reading and study of material in *Paramedic Care: Principles & Practice*, you notice any error or have any suggestions to improve either the textbook or workbook, please use the comment form at the back of this workbook. Alternatively, you can direct your comments via the Internet at the following address:

harrier@localnet.com

You can also visit the Brady website at:
www.bradybooks.com/paramedic

GUIDELINES TO BETTER TEST-TAKING

The knowledge you will gain from reading the textbook, completing the exercises in the workbook, listening in your paramedic class, and participating in your clinical and field experience will prepare you to care for patients who are seriously ill or injured. However, before you can practice these skills, you will have to pass several classroom written exams and your state's certification exam successfully. Your performance on these exams will depend not only on your knowledge but also on your ability to answer test questions correctly. The following guidelines are designed to help your performance on tests and to better demonstrate your knowledge of prehospital emergency care.

1. Relax and be calm during the test.

A test is designed to measure what you have learned and to tell you and your instructor how well you are doing. An exam is not designed to intimidate or punish you. Consider it a challenge, and just try to do your best. Get plenty of sleep prior to the examination. Avoid coffee or other stimulants for a few hours before the exam, and be prepared.

Reread the text chapters, review the objectives in the workbook, and review your class notes. It might be helpful to work with one or two other students and ask each other questions. This type of practice helps everyone better understand the knowledge presented in your course of study.

2. Read the questions carefully.

Read each word of the question and all the answers slowly. Words such as "except" or "not" may change the entire meaning of the question. If you miss such words, you may answer the question incorrectly even though you know the right answer.

EXAMPLE:
The art and science of Emergency Medical Services involves all of the following EXCEPT:

    A. sincerity and compassion
    B. respect for human dignity
    C. placing patient care before personal safety
    D. delivery of sophisticated emergency medical care
    E. none of the above

The correct answer is C, unless you miss the "EXCEPT."

3. Read each answer carefully.

Read each and every answer carefully. While the first answer may be absolutely correct, so may the rest, and thus the best answer might be "all of the above."

EXAMPLE:
Indirect medical control is considered to be:

    A. treatment protocols
    B. training and education
    C. quality assurance
    D. chart review
    E. all of the above

While answers A, B, C, and D are correct, the best and only acceptable answer is "all of the above," E.

4. Delay answering questions you don't understand and look for clues.

When a question seems confusing or you don't know the answer, note it on your answer sheet and come back to it later. This will ensure that you have time to complete the test. You will also find that other questions in the test may give you hints to answer the one you've skipped over. It will also prevent you from being frustrated with an early question and letting it affect your performance.

EXAMPLE:

Upon successful completion of a course of training as an EMT-P, most states will

    A. certify you (correct)
    B. license you
    C. register you
    D. recognize you as a paramedic
    E. issue you a permit

Another question, later in the exam, may suggest the right answer:

The action of one state in recognizing the certification of another is called:

    A. reciprocity (correct)
    B. national registration
    C. licensure
    D. registration
    E. extended practice

5. Answer all questions.

Even if you do not know the right answer, do not leave a question blank. A blank question is always wrong, while a guess might be correct. If you can eliminate some of the answers as wrong, do so. It will increase the chances of a correct guess.

EXAMPLE:

When a paramedic is called by the patient (through the dispatcher) to the scene of a medical emergency, the medical control physician has established a physician/patient relationship.

    A. True
    B. False

A true/false question gives you a 50 percent chance of a correct guess.

The hospital health professional responsible for sorting patients as they arrive at the emergency department is usually the:

    A. emergency physician
    B. ward clerk
    C. emergency nurse
    D. trauma surgeon
    E. A and C (correct)

A multiple-choice question with five answers gives a 20 percent chance of a correct guess. If you can eliminate one or more incorrect answers, you increase your odds of a correct guess to 25 percent, 33 percent, and so on. An unanswered question has a 0 percent chance of being correct.

Just before turning in your answer sheet, check to be sure that you have not left any items blank.

CHAPTER 1

The History

Review of Chapter Objectives

With each chapter of the Workbook, we identify the objectives and the important elements of the text content. You should review these items and refer to the pages listed if any points are not clear.

After reading this chapter, you should be able to:

1. Describe the techniques of history taking. pp. 5–11

For successful history taking, establish a rapport with the patient to gain his confidence and to set the stage for investigation of the chief complaint and medical history. Factors that will help in establishing rapport include:

- Well-groomed initial appearance
- Positive body language
- Good eye contact with the patient
- Professional demeanor
- Demonstration of interest in the patient

Your introduction should convey your interest in helping the patient and begin the two-way communication. It should convey your care and compassion for the patient and begin to build his trust in you.

Once you have introduced yourself and established your intent to help the patient, begin your questioning. Determine the formal chief complaint and investigate the current and past medical history. Pose questions in a way the patient understands, using terminology and the English language at the patient's level of comprehension.

Questioning frequently involves asking the patient personal, and possibly embarrassing, questions. At such times, ask these questions in a sensitive, nonthreatening way. "Ease into" the discussion of sensitive topics and use questions that are nonjudgmental. You may suggest to the patient that the issue of concern to him is common to many people in our society. Practice in questioning will help you develop the most effective approach. Be prepared to explain that the answers to questions are used for the patient's care and are not communicated beyond the necessary care providers.

2. Discuss the importance of using open- and closed-ended questions. p. 8

Open-ended questions allow the patient to explain or describe his or her symptoms or history in detail. This permits more complete and accurate patient answers and limits possible leading of patient responses.

Closed-ended questions limit patient responses to short answers—"yes" or "no," for example. Their use speeds information taking but the answers garnered elicit only limited information and may lead the patient toward answers.

During a complete patient history, use both types of questions to determine rapidly the nature and severity of the patient's problem and his medical history. Guide your questioning process by what the patient tells you, focusing on the possible medical problem, eliminating the least likely and identifying the most probable pathology.

3. Describe the use of, and differentiate among, facilitation, reflection, clarification, empathetic responses, confrontation, and interpretation. pp. 9–10

Facilitation is the support and encouragement of the patient as he explains his problem and answers your questions—for example, good eye contact, concerned facial expressions, leaning forward while listening.

Reflection is condensing and repeating what the patient says to guide patient response and encourage more focused answers.

Clarification is investigating a patient response by asking questions about it to garner further, more specific information.

Empathetic responses are facial expressions or statements like "I see" or "That must have been difficult" that display an understanding of, and a supportive feeling for, the patient's situation.

Confrontation is the questioning of a patient's responses when he appears to be denying or lying about the truth.

Interpretation is the use of the confrontation technique buttressed by the paramedic's suggestions, based on the evidence gathered to that point, of what the patient's problem may be.

4. Describe the structure, purpose, and how to obtain a comprehensive patient history. pp. 5–24

The comprehensive health history establishes a relationship between you and the patient and draws out pertinent information about the patient's medical history. This information may explain the current problem or guide further care in either the prehospital or in-hospital settings. The comprehensive patient history is gained by investigative questioning of the patient about past and current medical problems, including the chief complaint, the present illness (OPQRST-ASPN), the past medical history, current health status, and a review of systems.

5. List the components of a comprehensive history of an adult patient. pp. 11–19

The comprehensive patient history includes the following:

- Preliminary data (age, race, sex, etc.)
- The chief complaint
- The present illness or problem (including investigation of onset, provocation, quality, region/radiation, severity, time, as well as associated symptoms and pertinent negatives—OPQRST-ASPN)
- Past medical history (including the patient's general health, childhood and adult illnesses, psychiatric illness, serious accidents or injuries, and surgeries and hospitalizations)
- Current health status (including patient medications, allergies, use of tobacco, alcohol, and drugs, diet, recent screening tests and immunizations, exercise, leisure and sleep patterns, and environmental hazard/safety measures, family history, and psychosocial history)
- A review of systems (including, as appropriate, general physical information; skin; head, eyes, ears, nose, throat (HEENT); respiratory, cardiac; gastrointestinal; urinary; genital; peripheral vascular; musculoskeletal; neurologic; hematologic; endocrine; psychiatric)

The following objectives, while not listed in the chapter, will help in your understanding of the chapter content.

* Describe the review of systems and explain how it assists in identifying the patient's primary medical problem. pp. 17–19

The review of systems is an examination of each body system during the patient history. It is performed to rule out or further investigate medical problems and to assure that pertinent information is not overlooked during the assessment. Systems examined include:

- Skin
- Head, eyes, ears, nose, throat (HEENT)

- Respiratory
- Cardiac
- Gastrointestinal
- Urinary
- Genital
- Peripheral vascular
- Musculoskeletal
- Neurologic
- Hematologic
- Endocrine
- Psychiatric

* **Identify techniques for working with patients with special challenges.**   pp. 19–23

Silent patient. Be patient yourself. Speak reassuringly. Gently shake the patient. Consider a neurologic problem.

Overly talkative patient. Focus the patient on the important areas. Summarize what he or she says. Be patient.

Numerous symptoms. Be more clear in questioning; suspect an emotional problem.

Anxious patient. Encourage free conversation and reassure the patient.

Patient needing reassurance. Ask about his anxieties. Offer emotional support.

Anger and hostility. Accept the patient's responses without becoming defensive or angry.

Intoxicated patient. Be friendly and nonjudgmental. Listen to what the patient says, not how he says it. Make your safety and scene safety priorities.

Crying patient. Be patient. Accept the crying as a natural venting of emotions and be supportive.

Depression. Recognize the condition as a serious medical problem. Ask the patient whether he has had suicidal thoughts.

Sexually attractive or seductive patient. Maintain a professional relationship. Try to have a partner present.

Confusing behaviors or histories. Suspect mental illness, dementia, or delirium. Pay careful attention to the patient's mental status. Be reassuring.

Patient of limited intelligence. Try to evaluate the patient's mental abilities. Show genuine interest and establish a positive relationship. Elicit what information you can.

Language barriers. Seek out an interpreter. Be aware that important information is likely to be lost in translation.

Patient with hearing problems. Speak to the patient's best ear. If he reads lips, position yourself directly in front of him in good lighting, and speak slowly in a low-pitched voice. Consider writing your questions.

Patient who is blind or has limited vision. Identify yourself immediately and explain why you are there. Explain what you are doing before you do it.

Family and friends. If gaining pertinent information directly from the patient is difficult, talk to family members or friends on the scene.

CASE STUDY REVIEW

It is important to review each emergency response you participate in as a paramedic. Similarly, we will review the case study that precedes each chapter. We will address the important points of the response as addressed by the chapter. Often, this will include the scene size-up, patient assessment, patient management, patient packaging, and transport.

Reread the case study on pages 3 and 4 in Paramedic Care: Patient Assessment *and then read the discussion below.*

This case study draws attention to the value of the information gathered during the patient history and the process by which it is obtained.

The investigation of the chief complaint, associated symptoms, and the past medical history is extremely important both in determining what is wrong with your patient and then in guiding your provision of care. The circumstances of the emergency and the patient's presentation may confound you unless you employ a relatively standard, systematic approach to patient questioning, but one flexible enough to adapt to different circumstances. In a trauma emergency, you examine the mechanism of injury to determine what happened, while with a medical patient you must investigate the current and past medical history in depth.

Paramedic supervisor John Bigelow is presented with an "elderly man with abdominal pain." He begins his investigation of the history by introducing himself, identifying his role at the scene, and expressing his desire to help Mr. O'Donnell. He also asks for and uses Mr. O'Donnell's name to place the conversation on a more comfortable and personal level.

John first determines the patient's chief complaint, the problem that led him to call for the ambulance. (This may differ from the primary problem in some cases.) In this case, the chief complaint is, "My stomach hurts." John then quickly investigates the complaint by asking questions. The questions he asks are extensive and systematically examine the patient's symptoms. Note that these questions follow the acronym OPQRST-ASPN. John questions about Onset *(What were you doing when it started? Did it come on suddenly?)*, Provocation/Palliation *(Does anything make it better or worse?)*, Quality *(Can you describe how it feels?)*, Radiation *(Can you point to the area that hurts? Does the pain travel anywhere else?)*, Severity *(How bad is it? On a scale of ten, with ten being the worst pain you have ever felt, how would you rate this pain?)*, Time *(When did it start? Is it constant or does it come and go?)*, Associated Symptoms and Pertinent Negatives *(Are you nauseous and have you vomited? Have you experienced a change in your bowel habits? Do you have any difficulty breathing?)*. As John asks these questions, he leans forward and repeats parts of the patient's answers to show his interest and involvement.

The approach that John uses assures an ordered and in-depth investigation of all elements of the patient's history. At the emergency scene, there is much going on and often a sense of urgency. However, taking the few moments to inquire systematically about the patient's presentation assures that you have the essential information to begin forming a differential field diagnosis.

Based on what he has discovered, John begins to form his differential field diagnosis. While the history of pain right after eating and upper right quadrant pain suggest gall bladder problems (cholecystitis), John suspects a broader list of potential problems. This keeps him from forming tunnel vision. As he moves to investigate the past medical history, he asks questions to support or rule out these other problems.

John questions Mr. O'Donnell about his past medical history and gains further information about pain after eating fatty foods, indigestion, and alcohol consumption. The patient's denials of bloody emesis and stools are pertinent negatives that help John rule out other possible diagnoses. This information also helps him confirm a final field diagnosis of gall bladder problems. With the facts that support his evaluation, John conveys the results of his patient questioning to Dr. Zehner at the emergency department. The laboratory findings support the field diagnosis, and Mr. O'Donnell is quickly moved to surgery.

CONTENT SELF-EVALUATION

Each of the chapters in this Workbook includes a short content review. The questions are designed to test your ability to remember what you read. At the end of this Workbook, you can find the answers to the questions as well as the pages where the topic of the question was discussed in the text. If you answer the question incorrectly or are unsure of the answer, review the pages listed.

MULTIPLE CHOICE

1. In the majority of medical cases, the basis of the paramedic's field diagnosis is the:
   A. chief complaint
   B. index of suspicion
   C. mechanism of injury
   D. patient history
   E. vital signs

_A_ 2. Always accept information from previous caregivers gratefully, but briefly reconfirm it
with the patient.
    A. True
    B. False

_A_ 3. Elements of your patient questioning that will help you establish a trusting and professional relationship with the patient include all of the following EXCEPT:
    A. using medical terminology extensively
    B. making eye contact
    C. positioning yourself at the patient's eye level
    D. presenting a neat and clean appearance
    E. focusing your attention on the patient

_C_ 4. The list of possible causes for a patient's symptoms is the:
    A. index of suspicion
    B. mechanism of injury
    C. differential field diagnosis
    D. CAGE questionnaire
    E. nature of illness   *pg 5*

_A_ 5. It is appropriate, if not necessary, to take notes while interviewing the patient because it
is nearly impossible to remember everything important the patient tells you.
    A. True
    B. False

_C_ 6. Which of the following is an example of an open-ended question?
    A. Does your chest pain increase with breathing?
    B. Do you take diuretics?
    C. What does your pain feel like?
    D. Does the pain radiate to your shoulder?
    E. Have you had pain like this before?

_C_ 7. Which of the following questions is an example of a closed-ended question?
    A. What does your pain feel like?
    B. What were you doing when the pain started?
    C. Is your pain stabbing in nature?
    D. Why did you call us today?
    E. Where do you hurt?

_B_ 8. Always use a patient's first name during the interview to establish a closer, more trusting relationship.
    A. True   *pg 7*
    B. False

_____ 9. It is best to form a prearranged list of specific questions to assure you cover all bases
while interviewing your patient.
    A. True
    B. False

_B_ 10. The process of presenting the patient with an observation that he is hiding or masking
the truth is called:
    A. empathy
    B. confrontation
    C. reflection
    D. clarification
    E. facilitation

_B_ 11. The reason (pain, discomfort, or dysfunction) that the patient or other person summons
emergency medical services is termed the:
    A. primary problem
    B. chief complaint
    C. nature of the illness
    D. mechanism of injury
    E. none of the above   *pg 11-12*

_A_ **12.** The underlying cause of the patient's pain, discomfort, or dysfunction is called the:
  A. primary problem   **D.** mechanism of injury
  B. chief complaint   **E.** none of the above
  C. nature of the illness

_B_ **13.** Any activity that alleviates a patient's symptoms would fit under which element of the OPQRST–ASPN mnemonic for the history of the current illness?
  A. O   **D.** R
  B. P   **E.** S
  C. Q

_C_ **14.** Which of the following is an important part of the past medical history?
  A. radiation of the pain   **D.** quality of the pain
  B. last oral intake   **E.** all of the above
  C. surgeries or hospitalizations

_E_ **15.** A recently prescribed medication may account for medical problems due to which of the following?
  A. over-medication   **D.** untoward reaction
  B. under-medication   **E.** all of the above
  C. allergic reaction

_C_ **16.** Allergies should be expected for all of the following EXCEPT:
  A. the "caine" family   **D.** narcotics
  B. tetanus toxoid   **E.** both A and B
  C. glucose

_D_ **17.** A patient who has smoked 21 packs of cigarettes a week for 10 years has a pack history of:
  A. 21 pack/years   **D.** 30 pack/years
  B. 70 pack/years   **E.** 10 pack/years
  C. 7 pack/years

_B_ **18.** Which of the following is NOT a system examined during the review of systems?
  A. skin   **D.** hematologic system
  B. lymphatic system   **E.** endocrine system
  C. musculoskeletal system

_A_ **19.** Which step below would you attempt with the patient who suddenly goes silent?
  A. Stay calm and observe for nonverbal clues.
  B. Arrange for air medical transport.
  C. Terminate the interview immediately.
  D. Attempt to walk the patient back and forth a few times.
  E. Rapidly provide oral glucose.

_A_ **20.** Crying is a form of venting emotional stress; be patient and provide a patient who is crying with supportive remarks.
  A. True
  B. False

MATCHING

Write the letter of interview techniques in the space provided next to the appropriate description.

_C_ **21.** repeating the patient's words   **A.** empathy

_D_ **22.** using "go on" or "I'm listening"   **B.** confrontation

_E_ **23.** asking questions about patient's statements   **C.** reflection

_A_ **24.** showing you understand or feel for the patient **D.** facilitation

_B_ **25.** challenging a patient's statement   **E.** clarification

Classify each question or statement under the OPQRST category that best applies by writing the letter of the category in the space provided.

O. Onset
P. Provocation/palliation
Q. Quality
R. Region/radiation
S. Severity
T. Time

_S_ **26.** How does this compare to the worst pain you have ever felt?

_P_ **27.** Does rest lessen your pain?

_R_ **28.** Point to where you feel pain.

_Q_ **29.** Does this pain feel crushing in nature?

_P_ **30.** Does deep breathing increase the pain?

_O_ **31.** Did this pain begin suddenly or gradually?

_R_ **32.** Where does this pain travel to?

_T_ **33.** When did the first symptoms begin?

_Q_ **34.** Describe how the pain feels.

_P_ **35.** Were you walking or running when this pain first began?

SHORT ANSWER

36. Compare and contrast the differential field diagnosis and the final field diagnosis.

The differential field diagnosis is a list of possible causes for your patients symptoms throughout the assessment the final field diagnosis is what you have determined at the end of the assessment.

SPECIAL PROJECT

History of the Present Illness

Read the narrative description of a patient history below, and then organize the information into the OPQRST-ASPN format.

At just about noon, your unit, Rescue 31, responds to a "man down" call at a local park. You arrive to find a male, who appears to be in his early 20s, on the ground surrounded by onlookers. The man is sitting up and talking with a police officer. You introduce yourself and begin to form a general impression of the patient. He is an articulate male who seems conscious, alert, and fully oriented. The patient states that he was jogging when he suddenly had a sharp chest pain, became dizzy, and collapsed. He now complains of mild difficulty breathing and increased pain with deep breathing.

The patient states that the pain is very severe and ranks about 8 on a 1-to-10 scale, with 10 being the worst pain he ever experienced. He describes the pain as stabbing in nature and indicates its location, which is just to the left of the sternum at about the 3rd intercostal space. He denies pain anywhere else. The pain began suddenly, without warning, and he has never experienced anything like it. He denies taking a deep breath or coughing before the pain began. He says he has not had previous breathing or chest problems and says he does not have any history of COPD, asthma, or heart problems. He is not currently taking any medications nor is he being treated for any medical problem.

O. _Sudden_

P. _He was jogging / He collapsed / increased pain c̄ deep breathing_

Q. _Sharp Chest Pain, mild SOB, stabbing in nature._

R. _to the left of the Sternum, about the third intercostal space._

S. _Very severe, 8:10 on a 1-10 scale_

T. _About noon, sudden_

AS. _Dizzy, collapsed, Difficulty breathing_

PN. _No prev. breathing or chest problems, Ø Hx COPD, asthma, Ø medications, Ø prev. Med Tx._

CHAPTER 2

*

Physical Exam Techniques

Because Chapter 2 is lengthy, it has been divided into sections to aid your study. Read the assigned text pages, then progress through the objectives and self-evaluation materials as you would with other chapters. When you feel secure in your grasp of the content, proceed to the next section.

Section I, pp. 27–77

Review of Chapter Objectives

After reading this chapter, you should be able to:

1. **Define and describe the techniques of inspection, palpation, percussion, and auscultation.**   pp. 29–33

   Inspection is the process of informed observation, viewing the patient for anatomical shape, coloration, and movement. It is the least invasive examination tool, yet may provide the most patient information.

   Palpation is the use of touch to gather information regarding size, shape, position, temperature, moisture, texture, movement, and response to pressure. The fingertips are most sensitive, while the palm best evaluates vibration and the back of the hand, temperature.

   Percussion is the production of a vibration in tissue to elicit sounds. These sounds—dull, resonant, hyperresonant, tympanic, and flat—identify the nature of the tissue underneath. The vibration is generated by striking the first knuckle of a finger placed against the area to be percussed with the fingertip of the other hand.

   Auscultation is listening for sounds within the body, most frequently with a stethoscope. The intensity, pitch, duration, quality, and timing of sounds in the patient's lungs, heart, blood vessels, and intestines are compared against normal sounds.

3. **Evaluate the importance of a general survey.**   pp. 41–48

   The general survey is the first part of the comprehensive exam. It is made up of your evaluation of the patient's appearance—including level of consciousness, expression, state of health, general characteristics (weight, height, etc.), posturing, dress, grooming, etc.—the vital signs, and additional assessments such as pulse oximetry, cardiac monitoring, and blood glucose determination. The survey helps you form a general impression of your patient's health.

4. **Describe the examination of the following body regions, differentiate between normal and abnormal findings, and define the significance of abnormal findings:**

   Skin, hair, and nails   pp. 49–57
   Observe the skin carefully for color, especially in the nail beds, lips, conjunctiva, and mucous membranes of the mouth. Pink skin reflects good oxygenation, while pale skin reflects poor blood

flow from hypovolemia, hypothermia, compensatory shock, or anemia. A bluish-colored skin, cyanosis, suggests blood is low in oxygen. A yellow sclera or general discoloration, jaundice, is due to liver failure. Other skin observations may include petechiae, small round, flat purplish spots caused by capillary bleeding from a variety of etiologies, and ecchymosis, a larger, black-and-blue discoloration that is often the result of trauma or bleeding disorders. Moisture, temperature, texture, mobility, and turgor are also evaluated. Skin lesions are disruptions in normal tissue that may take on almost any shape, color, or arrangement.

Inspect and palpate the hair to determine color, quality, distribution, quantity, and texture and inspect and palpate the scalp for scaling, lesions, redness, lumps, or tenderness. Generalized hair loss may reflect chemotherapy; failure to develop normal hair patterns may be caused by a pituitary or hormonal problem; and unusual facial hair in women suggests a hormonal imbalance. Mild scalp flaking suggests dandruff; heavy scaling, psoriasis; and greasy scaling, seborrheic dermatitis. Lice eggs (nits) may be found firmly attached to the hair shafts. Normal hair texture is smooth and soft in Caucasians; in people of African descent, the texture is coarser. Dry, brittle, or fragile hair is abnormal.

Inspect the finger and toenails for color. Note any discolorations, lesions, ridging, grooves, depressions, or pitting. Depressions suggest systemic disease. Compress the nail and bed to determine its adherence and look for nail hygiene. Any boggyness suggests cardiorespiratory disease.

Head, scalp, and skull   pp. 57–59, 62
Observe and palpate the skull and facial region for symmetry, smoothness, wounds, bleeding, size, and general contour. Examine the hair and scalp as described above. Check the eyes for bilateral periorbital and mastoid ecchymosis, "raccoon eyes" and "Battle's sign," respectively. They suggest basilar skull fracture and occur an hour or so after injury. Palpate the facial region for crepitation, false motion, or instability suggesting fracture. Evaluate the temporomandibular joint for pain, tenderness, swelling, and range of motion. Have the patient open and close his mouth and jut and retract his jaw. Any loss of normal function suggests injury.

Eyes, ears, nose, mouth, and pharynx   pp. 59–74
Examine for visual acuity as described below (objective 5), then evaluate for peripheral vision. While the patient faces you, have him look at your nose while you extend your arms, bend your elbows and wiggle the fingers. If he notices the fingers moving in all four directions (up, down, left, and right) for each eye, his peripheral vision is grossly normal. Inspect the eyes for symmetry, shape, inflammation, swelling, misalignment (disconjugate gaze), lesions, and contour. Examine the eyelids, open and closed, for swelling, discoloration, droop (ptosis), styes, and lash positioning. Observe the tearing or dryness of the eyes. Gently retract the lower eyelid while asking the patient to look through a range of motion. Examine the sclera for signs of irritation, cloudiness, yellow discoloration (jaundice), any nodules, swelling, discharge, or hemorrhage into the scleral tissue. With an oblique light source, inspect the cornea for opacities. Inspect the size, shape, symmetry, and reactivity of the pupils. Note the pupils' direct and consensual response to increased light intensity. A sluggish pupil suggests pressure on CN-III; bilateral sluggishness suggests global hypoxia or depressant drug action. Constricted pupils suggest opiate overdose, while dilated and fixed pupils reflect brain anoxia. Ask the patient to focus on your finger close at hand, then move the hand to his nose, then away. The eyes should converge, while the pupils should constrict slightly. Then have him follow your finger as you move it through an "H" pattern. The eyes should move smoothly together. Nystagmus is a jerky movement at the distal extremes of ocular movement. Gently touch the cornea with a strand of cotton. The patient should respond with a blink. Using an ophthalmoscope, look into the eye's anterior chamber for signs of blood (hyphema), cells, or pus (hypopyon), and check the cornea for lacerations, abrasions, cataracts, papilledema (from increased ICP), vascular occlusions, and retinal hemorrhage.

Examine the ears by looking for symmetry from in front of the patient, then examine each ear separately. Examine the external portion (auricle) for shape, size, landmarks, and position on the head. Examine the surrounding area for deformities, lesions, tenderness, and erythema. Pull the helix upward and outward, press on the tragus and on the mastoid process and note any discomfort or pain suggesting otitis or mastoiditis. Some pain may be associated with toothache, a cold, sore throat, or cervical spine injury. Inspect the ear canal for discharge (pus, mucus, blood, or cerebral spinal fluid [CSF]) and inflammation. Trauma can account for blood, mucus, and CSF in the ear canal. Check hearing acuity by covering one ear and whispering, then speaking into the other. Hearing loss may be accounted for by trauma, accumulation of debris (often cerumen), tympanic membrane rupture, drug use, and prolonged exposure to loud noise. Visualize the inner canal with the otoscope. With the largest speculum that will fit the canal, turn the patient's head away from you, pull the auricle slightly up and backward, and insert the otoscope. Inspect for wax (cerumen), discharge, redness, lesions, perforations, and foreign bodies. Then focus on the tympanic membrane. It should be a translucent pearly gray. Color changes suggest fluid behind the eardrum or infection. Also check for bulging, protractions, or perforations.

Visualize the patient's nose from the front and sides to determine any asymmetry, deviation, tenderness, flaring, or abnormal color. Tilt your patient's head back slightly and examine the nostrils. Insert the otoscope and check for deviation of the septum and perforations. Examine the nasal mucosa for color, and the color, consistency, and quantity of drainage. Rhinitis (a runny nose) suggests seasonal allergies; a thick yellow discharge, infection; and blood, epistaxis from trauma or a septal defect. Test each side of the nose for patency by occluding the other side during a breath. There is normally some difference in patency between the sides. Palpate the frontal sinuses for swelling and tenderness.

Begin assessment of the mouth by observing the lips for color and condition. They should be pink, smooth, symmetrical, and without lesions, swelling, lumps, cracks, or scaliness. Using a bright light and tongue blade, examine the oral mucosa for color, lesions, white patches, or fissures. The mucosa should be pinkish-red, smooth, and moist. The gums should be pink with clearly defined margins around the teeth. The teeth should be well formed and straight. If the gums are swollen, bleed easily, and are separated from the teeth, suspect periodontal disease. Ask the patient to stick his tongue out and note its velvety surface. Hold the tongue with a 2" × 2" gauze pad and inspect all sides and the bottom. All surfaces should be pink and smooth. Then examine the pharynx and have the patient say "aaaahhh" while you hold the tongue down with a tongue blade. Watch the movement of the uvula and the coloration and condition of the palatine tonsils and posterior pharynx. Look for any pus, swelling, ulcers, or drainage. Also notice any odors including alcohol, feces (bowel obstruction), acetone (diabetic ketoacidosis), gastric contents, coffee-grounds-like material (gastric hemorrhage), pink-tinged sputum (pulmonary edema), or the smell of bitter almonds (cyanide poisoning).

Neck   **pp. 74–77**

Inspect your patient's neck for symmetry and visible masses. Note any deformity, deviations, tugging, scars, gland enlargement, or visible lymph nodes. Examine for any open wounds and cover them with an occlusive dressing. Examine the jugular veins for distention while the patient is seated upright and at a 45° incline. Palpate the trachea to assure it is inline. Palpate the thyroid while the patient swallows to assure it is small, smooth, and without nodules. Palpate each lymph node to determine size, shape, tenderness, consistency, and mobility. Tender, swollen, and mobile nodes suggest inflammation from infection, while hard and fixed ones suggest malignancy.

5. **Describe the assessment of visual acuity.**   **pp. 60–61**

Visual acuity is the ability to read detail. A wall chart with lines of progressively smaller letters is placed at 20 feet from the patient. He then reads to the smallest line in which he can recognize at least one half the letters. The result is recorded as the distance from the chart and the distance at which a person with normal sight could distinguish the letters, 20/20 for normal or 20/60 for someone who reads what is normally read at 60 feet.

6. **Explain the rationale for the use of an ophthalmoscope and otoscope.**   **pp. 39, 65–67**

The ophthalmoscope is a light source and a series of lenses that permit you to examine the interior of the patient's eyes. It allows you to examine the retina, blood vessels, and optic nerve at the back of the posterior chamber of the eye.

The otoscope is a light source and a magnifying lens that permits examination of a patient's ears and nose. It allows you to examine the external auditory canal and the tympanic membrane for trauma, irritation, or infection.

8. Describe percussion of the chest.

pp. 79, 83

Percuss both the anterior and posterior chest surfaces, examining for resonant (normal), hyper-resonant (air-filled pneumothorax or tension pneumothorax) or dull sounds. Percuss both sides symmetrically from the apex to the base at 5 centimeter intervals, avoiding the scapulae. Determine the boundaries of any hyperresonance or dullness.

9. Differentiate the percussion notes and their characteristics.

pp. 31–32

Percussion provides three basic sounds; dull, resonant, and hyperresonant. Dull reflects a density and is a medium-pitched thud. It is usually caused by a dense organ (like the liver) or fluid, like blood, underneath. Resonant sounds are generally associated with a less dense tissue, like the lungs, and are lower-pitched and longer lasting sounds. Hyperresonant sounds reflect air, or air under pressure, and are the lowest-pitched sounds and the ones that diminish in volume most slowly.

The following objectives, while not listed in the chapter, will help in your understanding of the chapter content.

* Identify and describe the vital signs.

pp. 33–37

Pulse is the wave of pressure generated by the heart as it expels blood into the arterial system. It is measured by palpating a distal artery (or auscultated during blood pressure determination) and is evaluated for rate, rhythm, and quality (strength). The normal pulse is strong, regular, and has a rate of between 60 and 80 beats per minute.

Respiration is the movement of air through the airway and into and out of the lungs. It is evaluated by observing and/or feeling chest excursion and listening to air movement. The rate, effort, and quality (depth and pattern) of respirations are determined. Normal respiration moves a tidal volume of 500 mL at a rate of 12 to 20 times per minute with symmetrical chest wall movement.

Blood pressure is the force of blood against the arterial wall during the cardiac/pulse cycle. It is measured using a sphygmomanometer (blood pressure cuff) and stethoscope. The maximum or systolic blood pressure—the reading obtained when the ventricles contract, the lower or diastolic blood pressure—the reading obtained when the ventricles relax, and the difference between them, the pulse pressure, are evaluated. The systolic pressure is usually between 100 and 135, and the diastolic, between 60 and 80.

Temperature is the body core temperature and is the product of heat-creating metabolism and body heat loss. It is measured by a glass or electronic thermometer placed in the axilla, mouth, or rectum. Normal body temperature is 98.6°F (37°C).

* Identify and explain the importance of additional assessment techniques.

pp. 46–48

Pulse oximetry is the noninvasive measurement of oxygen saturation in the tissue of a distal extremity. It provides a real-time evaluation of oxygen delivery to the distal circulation. Normal readings are between 96 and 100 percent. Readings below this reflect problems with either respiration or circulation and demand intervention.

Cardiac monitoring uses electronics to display the electrical activity of the heart. The monitor shows an electronic or paper tracing of the heart's activity, either a normal rhythm, a dysrhythmia, or no activity—asystole. This information is essential to identifying when to shock the heart back to a normal rhythm or to treat it through the use of medication.

Blood glucose determination is performed by using a glucometer, a small electronic device that evaluates the color of a blood-stained reagent strip. The glucose level can rule out or identify hypoglycemia in a patient with a lowered level of consciousness or in the known diabetic.

CASE STUDY REVIEW

Reread the case study on pages 27 and 28 in Paramedic Care: Patient Assessment *before reading the discussion below.*

This case study clearly shows the benefit of a planned and well-directed physical examination of a patient with nonspecific signs and symptoms of disease. Here, Dale and Pam use the assessment to search out the possible causes, then converge, through specific signs and symptoms, on the patient's problem, their field diagnosis.

Dale and Pam arrive to care for a patient with very confusing and nonspecific signs and symptoms of illness. They and their patient, Mr. Dalton, count heavily on the comprehensive physical assessment to help sort out what might be wrong. A case like this is one of the few times you, as a paramedic, will employ most of the elements of a complete and detailed physical exam. More frequently you will quickly identify the likely causes of your patient's chief complaint and presenting signs and symptoms—a differential diagnosis. Then you will focus your assessment on evaluating the presenting signs and symptoms and looking for those commonly associated with the diseases you suspect. This information then helps you rule out or support a problem, arriving at a single suspected problem, the field diagnosis.

Dale and Pam perform a quick initial assessment to evaluate Mr. Dalton's mental status and ABCs. His first few words demonstrate that he is conscious and alert, and his airway and breathing are more than adequate. His mental status suggests his brain is being well perfused and a quick pulse check confirms good circulation. With the elements of the initial assessment complete, Dale and Pam move to the focused history and physical exam without a clear idea of what might be affecting Mr. Dalton.

Since Mr. Dalton's presentation is nonspecific to a particular medical problem, they must use the focused history and physical exam to investigate his physical and mental state more carefully. Elements of the patient history begin to direct their investigation toward a vascular problem—a history of coronary artery disease, hypertension, and the use of certain medications—nitroglycerin, aspirin, and digoxin. *(Through his training and experience, Dale knows that nitroglycerin is given to reduce the demands on a heart with limited perfusion, that aspirin is used to reduce the risk of clot development, and that digoxin is often given for atrial fibrillation, which is frequently associated with pulmonary and cerebral emboli.)* Added to the physical assessment finding—general weakness and an unstable walk and stance—what Dale and Pam learn suggests some motor or neurologic problem.

The team takes a quick set of vital signs that reveal only an abnormally high blood pressure, which is consistent with the history of hypertension. Dale performs the elements of the general survey and examines Mr. Dalton's appearance, level of consciousness, signs of distress, state of health, vital statistics, sexual development, skin color and lesions, posture, gait and motor activity, dress, grooming and personal hygiene, body or breath odor, and facial expression. They reveal a patient in generally good health with an appropriate affect. The only noted problem is one of coordinated walking (gait). The detailed physical exam reflects spasms at the outer reaches of left lateral eye movement, nystagmus. This coupled with the gait problem suggests a neurologic problem for which Dale begins a complete neurologic examination.

Dale investigates posture, balance, reflexes, and coordination. Clearly Mr. Dalton is slumped to the left side. Dale finds balance problems with Mr. Dalton, no doubt, drifting to the left when his eyes are closed. His reflexes are normal, at least for a 70-year-old man. His complaint about buttoning his shirt suggests a coordination problem, which Dale investigates further. He employs a few repetitive action exercises (thumb touch, shin touch, and palm-up/palm-down to thigh) that reveal a clear neurologic deficit on Mr. Dalton's left side.

Because of the left-sided slumping, nystagmus, and impaired coordination, Dale concludes that this is a cerebellar problem, most likely due to an arterial blockage. This is supported by both the history of earlier, less significant events (possibly transient ischemic events and an evolving stroke) and the vascular disease history discovered earlier. Note that motor and sensory function is controlled by the contralateral side of the brain (cerebral injury) and coordination is controlled by the ipsilateral cerebellum.

In this scenario, Dale and Pam would also be likely to apply the cardiac monitor and evaluate the ECG for dysrhythmia. They might also auscultate the carotid arteries for bruit, suggestive of vascular disease that may be the origin of an emboli. In some EMS systems, stroke patients may be given clot-busting drugs like TPA or streptokinase to dissolve blockage and reduce the effects of the infarct. In such a system, Dale and Pam may have a series of questions to ask of Mr. Dalton to rule out the risk of internal hemorrhage, to help specifically identify the type of stroke or cerebrovascular accident, and to reduce the time from infarct to medication.

CONTENT SELF-EVALUATION

MULTIPLE CHOICE

1. Of the physical examination techniques used in prehospital care, which is the least invasive?
    A. inspection
    B. auscultation
    C. palpation
    D. percussion
    E. C and D

2. "Crackles" would be found using which of the following assessment techniques?
    A. palpation
    B. auscultation
    C. inspection
    D. percussion
    E. none of the above

3. "Guarding" would be discovered using which of the following assessment techniques?
    A. palpation
    B. auscultation
    C. inspection
    D. percussion
    E. none of the above

4. Which of the following techniques should be performed first during the physical examination?
    A. palpation
    B. auscultation
    C. inspection
    D. percussion
    E. none of the above

5. Which part of the hands and fingers is best suited to evaluate tissue consistency?
    A. tips of the fingers
    B. pads of the fingers
    C. palm of the hand
    D. back of the hands or fingers
    E. none of the above

6. Which part of the hands and fingers is best suited to evaluate vibration?
    A. tips of the fingers
    B. pads of the fingers
    C. palm of the hand
    D. back of the hands or fingers
    E. none of the above

7. Noticing areas of warmth during palpation might reflect an injury before significant edema and discoloration develop.
    A. True
    B. False

8. The booming sound produced by percussing an air-filled region is:
    A. hyperresonance
    B. dull
    C. resonance
    D. flat
    E. none of the above

9. The only region where you perform auscultation as other than the last step of assessment is the:
    A. anterior thorax
    B. neck
    C. abdomen
    D. peripheral arteries
    E. posterior thorax

_B_ 10. A heart rate above 100 is known as a:
- A. bradycardia
- B. tachycardia
- C. hypercardia
- D. tachypnea
- E. bradypnea

_E_ 11. One likely cause of bradycardia is:
- A. fever
- B. pain
- C. parasympathetic stimulation
- D. fear
- E. blood loss

_A_ 12. Which of the following is NOT an aspect of pulse evaluation?
- A. volume
- B. rhythm
- C. quality
- D. rate
- E. none of the above

_E_ 13. Normal exhalation is:
- A. an active process involving accessory muscles
- B. an active process involving the diaphragm and intercostal muscles
- C. active in its early stages and passive in later stages
- D. passive in its early stages and active in later stages
- E. a passive process

_A_ 14. For a patient with an airway obstruction, exhalation is likely to be:
- A. an active process involving accessory muscles
- B. an active process involving only the diaphragm and intercostal muscles
- C. active in its early stages and passive in later stages
- D. passive in its early stages and active in later stages
- E. a passive process

_D_ 15. The amount of air a patient moves into and out of his lungs in one breath is the:
- A. normal volume
- B. respiratory volume
- C. residual volume
- D. tidal volume
- E. minute volume

_D_ 16. The pressure of the blood within the blood vessels while the ventricles are relaxing is the:
- A. Korotkoff blood pressure
- B. systolic blood pressure
- C. diastolic blood pressure
- D. asystolic blood pressure
- E. atrial blood pressure

_A_ 17. The diastolic blood pressure represents a measure of:
- A. systemic vascular resistance
- B. the cardiac output
- C. the viscosity of the blood
- D. the strength of ventricular contraction
- E. relative blood volume

_E_ 18. Which of the following are likely to influence a patient's blood pressure?
- A. anxiety
- B. position (lying, sitting, standing)
- C. recent smoking
- D. eating
- E. all of the above

_C_ 19. Generally, hypertension in a healthy adult is any blood pressure higher than:
- A. 120/80
- B. 140/90
- C. 160/90
- D. 180/100
- E. 200/100

_C_ 20. What is the pulse pressure in a patient with the following vital signs: pulse 82 and strong; respirations 14 and full: and blood pressure 144/96?
- A. 14
- B. 40
- C. 48
- D. 96
- E. 120

_____ 21. In the tilt test, what vital sign change is a positive sign of hypovolemia?
A. blood pressure drops by 10 to 20 mmHg
B. blood pressure rises by 10 to 20 mmHg
C. pulse rate drops by 10 to 20 beats per minute
D. pulse rate rises by 10 to 20 beats per minute
E. either A or D

_____ 22. Hyperthermia can result from all of the following EXCEPT:
A. high environmental temperatures
B. infections
C. reduced metabolic activity
D. drugs
E. increases in metabolic activity

_____ 23. What technique of stethoscope use best transmits low-pitched sound to the ear?
A. light pressure on the diaphragm
B. firm pressure on the diaphragm
C. moderate pressure on the bell
D. light pressure on the bell
E. strong pressure on the bell

_____ 24. The bell of a stethoscope is best for listening to the sounds of:
A. blood vessel bruits
B. the blood pressure
C. the heart
D. the lung
E. none of the above

_____ 25. Which of the following is NOT a characteristic of a good stethoscope?
A. thick, heavy tubing
B. long tubing (70 to 100 cm)
C. snug-fitting earpieces
D. a bell with a rubber-ring edge
E. all of the above

_____ 26. Generally, each narrow line on a sphygmomanometer represents what pressure difference?
A. 1 mmHg
B. 2 mmHg
C. 4 mmHg
D. 5 mmHg
E. 10 mmHg

_____ 27. If a patient has a regular and strong pulse, you should determine the pulse rate by assessing the number of beats in:
A. two minutes and dividing by 2
B. three minutes
C. 30 seconds and multiplying by 2
D. 15 seconds and multiplying by 4
E. 10 seconds and multiplying by 5

_____ 28. Use of which of the following pulse points is recommended with a small child?
A. radial
B. brachial
C. carotid
D. popliteal
E. dorsalis pedis

_____ 29. It is important to attempt to evaluate your patient's respiratory rate and volume without his being aware of it.
A. True
B. False

_____ 30. The proper position of the patient's arm when taking the blood pressure is:
A. arm slightly flexed
B. palm up
C. fingers relaxed
D. clothing removed from the upper arm
E. all of the above

_____ 31. The sphygmomanometer should be inflated to what level beyond the point at which the patient's radial pulse disappears?
A. 10 mmHg
B. 20 mmHg
C. 30 mmHg
D. 40 mmHg
E. between B and C

_____ 32. The first blood pressure reading is the systolic blood pressure, indicated by the early deflections of the sphygmomanometer needle.
   A. True
   B. False

_____ 33. When using the oral glass thermometer, it should be left in the mouth for what period of time?
   A. 30 to 45 seconds
   B. 30 to 60 seconds
   C. 1 to 2 minutes
   D. 2 minutes
   E. 3 to 4 minutes

_____ 34. The normal patient oxygen saturation without supplemental oxygen at sea level should be:
   A. between 90 to 95 percent
   B. below 95 percent
   C. 100 percent
   D. 96 to 100 percent
   E. below 90 percent

_____ 35. A patient suffering from carbon monoxide poisoning will likely have a pulse oximetry reading that is:
   A. accurate
   B. falsely high
   C. falsely low
   D. erratic and inaccurate
   E. unreadable

_____ 36. The ECG of a cardiac monitor can tell you all of the following EXCEPT:
   A. the heart rate
   B. the sequence of cardiac events
   C. the timing of cardiac events
   D. the pumping ability of the heart
   E. A and C above

_____ 37. The skin regulates body temperature through:
   A. radiation
   B. evaporation
   C. conduction
   D. convection
   E. all of the above

_____ 38. Pale skin is least likely to be caused by which of the following?
   A. increased deoxyhemoglobin
   B. a cold environment
   C. shock compensation
   D. anemia
   E. hypovolemic shock

_____ 39. Which of the following skin discolorations represents a yellow hue?
   A. cyanosis
   B. jaundice
   C. eccyhmosis
   D. erythema
   E. pallor

_____ 40. A heavy scaling of the skin under the hair is:
   A. dandruff
   B. nits
   C. seborrheic dermatitis
   D. psoriasis
   E. none of the above

_____ 41. With age, the toenails are likely to become:
   A. hard
   B. thick
   C. brittle
   D. yellowish
   E. all of the above

_____ 42. The blueish discoloration around the orbits of the eyes, suggestive of a basilar skull fracture, is called:
   A. "racoon eyes"
   B. "Battle's sign"
   C. periorbital ecchymosis
   D. retroauricular ecchymosis
   E. either A or C

_____ 43. The cranial nerves that control eye movement are:
A. I, II, and III
B. II, III, and IV
C. III, IV, and VI
D. II, VI, and VII
E. V, VI, and VIII

_____ 44. The muscular and colored portion of the eye that constricts and dilates to regulate light falling on the retinal surface is the:
A. retina
B. pupil
C. conjunctiva
D. iris
E. lens

_____ 45. The characteristic of the unaffected eye responding to stimuli in the affected eye is:
A. consenual response
B. direct response
C. simultaneous response
D. ipsilateral response
E. none of the above

_____ 46. About 20 percent of the population have a noticeable difference in the size of the pupils, a condition called:
A. hyphema
B. anisocoria
C. glaucoma
D. hypopyon
E. none of the above

_____ 47. The ear provides what important body function beyond hearing?
A. equalization of pressure during yawning
B. vibration sensation
C. balance and head position sense
D. equalization of body and outside pressure
E. all of the above except B

_____ 48. Otorrhea is a discharge from the ear that may contain:
A. pus
B. mucus
C. blood
D. cerebrospinal fluid
E. all of the above

_____ 49. The term for a common nosebleed is:
A. epistaxis
B. otorrhea
C. rhinorrhea
D. rhinitis
E. none of the above

_____ 50. The most superior and prominent airway structure in the neck is the:
A. cricoid cartilage
B. thyroid cartilage
C. tracheal ring
D. thyroid gland
E. jugular vein

SPECIAL PROJECT

Vital Signs

For each of the following vital signs, list the normal range of values and any other important considerations in their evaluation.

Pulse:

_____

_____

_____

Respirations:

_____

_____

_____

_____

_____

_____

_____

Blood pressure:

_____

_____

_____

_____

_____

_____

_____

_____

Temperature:

_____

_____

_____

_____

_____

_____

_____

_____

CHAPTER 2

Physical Exam Techniques

Section II, pp. 77–127

Review of Chapter Objectives

After reading this chapter, you should be able to:

4. **Describe the examination of the following body regions, differentiate between normal and abnormal findings, and define the significance of abnormal findings:**

    Thorax (anterior and posterior)   **pp. 77–83**

    To assess the chest, you need a stethoscope with a bell and diaphragm. Expose the entire thorax with consideration for the patient's dignity and modesty, and inspect, palpate, percuss, and auscultate. Compare findings from one side of the chest to the other and from posterior to anterior. Look for general shape and symmetry as well as for the rate and pattern of breathing. Observe for retractions and the use of accessory muscles (suggestive of airway obstruction or restriction), and palpate for deformities, tenderness, crepitus (suggestive of rib fracture), and abnormal chest excursion (suggestive of flail chest or spinal injury). Feel for vibrations associated with air movement and speech. Percuss the chest for dullness (hemothorax, pleural effusion, or pneumonia), resonance, and hyperresonance (pneumothorax or tension pneumothorax). Finally, auscultate the lung lobes for normal breath sounds, crackles (pulmonary edema), wheezes (asthma), rhonchi, stridor (airway obstruction), and pleural friction rubs.

    Arterial pulse including rate, rhythm, and amplitude   **pp. 86–88**

    Locate a soft and pulsing carotid artery in the neck, just lateral to the cricoid cartilage to avoid pressure on the carotid sinus. Carefully press down until the pulse wave just lifts your finger off the artery. Determine the rate and carefully evaluate for regularity. Irregularity may be caused by dysrhythmia, while variation in strength may be due to such phenomena as pulsus paradoxus, increasing strength with exhalation and decreasing with inhalation. Also note any thrills (humming or vibration) and listen with the stethoscope for bruits (sounds of turbulent flow).

    Jugular venous pressure and pulsations   **pp. 86–88**

    Examine the anterior neck and locate the jugular veins. Position your patient with his head elevated 30° and turned away from you. Look for pulsation just above the suprasternal notch. Identify the highest point of pulsation and measure the distance from the sternal angle. The highest point of pulsation is usually between 1 and 2 cm from the sternal angle. (Distension when the patient is elevated at higher angles may reflect tension pneumothorax or pericardial tamponade, while flat veins at lower angles may suggest hypovolemia.)

    Abdomen   **pp. 89–97**

    Question your patient regarding any pain, tenderness or unusual feeling, and recent bowel and bladder function. Carefully inspect the area for scars, dilated veins, stretch marks, rashes, lesions, and pigmentation changes. Discoloration around the umbilicus (Cullen's sign) or over the flanks (Grey-Turner's sign) suggest intra-abdominal hemorrhage. Assess the size and shape of the abdomen, determining whether it is scaphoid (concave), flat, round, or distended, and look for any bulges or hernias. Ascites result in bulges in the flanks and across the abdomen suggesting congestive heart or liver failure, while suprapubic bulges suggest a full bladder or pregnant uterus. Look also for any masses, palpations, or peristalsis. A slight vascular pulsing is normal, but excessive movement suggests an aneurysm. Auscultate and percuss as described earlier. Then depress each quadrant gently and release. Look for patient expression or muscle guarding suggestive of injury or peritonitis.

Male and female genitalia   pp. 95–99

Assure patient privacy, a warm environment, and patient modesty during the exam; also be sure the patient has emptied his or her bladder before beginning. Expose only those body areas that you must, and explain what you are going to do before you do it. Inspect the genitalia for development and maturity. Visually inspect the mons pubis, labia, and perineum of the female patient for swelling, lesions, or irritation suggestive of a sebaceous cyst or sexually transmitted disease. Check the hair bases for small red maculopapules suggestive of lice. Retract the labia and inspect the inner labia and urethral opening. Examine for a white curdy discharge (fungal infection) or yellow-green discharge (bacterial infection). For the male, inspect the penis and testicles, noting inflammation and lesions suggestive of sexually transmitted disease. Check for lice and examine the glans for degeneration, inflammation, or discharge. Yellow discharge is reflective of gonorrhea.

Anus and rectum   pp. 99–100

Position your patient on his or her left side with legs flexed and buttocks near the edge of the stretcher. Be sensitive to the patient's feelings and drape or cover any areas not being observed. With a gloved hand, spread the buttocks apart and examine the area for lumps, ulcers, inflammations, rashes, or lesions. Palpate any areas carefully, noting inflammation or tenderness. If appropriate, obtain a fecal sample for testing.

Musculoskeletal system   pp. 100–127

Advancing age causes changes in the musculoskeletal system including shortening and increased curvature of the spine, a reduction in muscle mass and strength, and a reduction in the range of motion. Observe the patient's general posture, build, and muscular development as well as the movement of the extremities, gait, and position at rest. Then inspect all regions of the body for deformities, symmetry and symmetrical movement, joint structure, and swelling, nodules, or inflammation. Deformities are often related to misaligned articulating bones, dislocations, or subluxations. Impaired movement is usually related to arthritis; nodules related to rheumatic fever or rheumatoid arthritis; and redness related to gout, rheumatic fever, or arthritis. Compare dissimilar joints to determine what structures might be affected. Assess range of motion by moving the limb, ask the patient to move the limb, and then ask the patient to move the limb against resistance. Note any asymmetry and inequality between active and passive motion. Also examine for crepitation (a grating vibration or sound) that may suggest arthritis, an inflamed joint, or a fracture. Avoid manipulating a deformed or painful joint. Perform a physical exam on each joint, moving it through its normal range of motion and noting any deformities, limited or resistant movement, tenderness, and swelling.

7. Describe the survey of respiration.   pp. 34–36, 79–83

The survey of the chest assesses the thorax and respiration by inspection, palpation, percussion, and auscultation. Compare findings side to side and anterior to back. Visualize and auscultate the five lung lobes during your exam. Examine the patient's respiration, looking for increased inspiratory or expiratory time or any sounds indicating upper or lower airway obstruction. Examine the chest for symmetry and symmetry of motion and any retraction or any anterior-posterior dimension abnormality. Also feel for any unusual vibrations associated with speech. Percuss the chest and note any hyperresonance or dullness. Listen through the stethoscope for lung sounds over each lobe and note any crackles or wheezes. Identify the respiratory rate and volume of each breath and determine the minute volume.

10. **Describe special examination techniques related to the assessment of the chest.** pp. 77–83

Chest excursion
Place your hands with the fingers spread at the 10th intercostal space and feel for chest excursion as the patient breathes deeply. Your hand should move equally about 3 to 5 cm with each breath.

Fremitus
Place a cupped hand against the chest wall at various locations and feel for vibrations while the patient says "ninety-nine" or "one-on-one." These vibrations should be equal throughout the chest. Note any enhanced, decreased, or absent fremitus.

Diaphragm excursion
Percuss the border of the rib cage for the dullness of the diaphragm during quiet breathing. Then mark the highest and lowest movement during respiration. Repeat the process on the other side of the chest. This excursion should be about 6 cm and equal on each side.

11. **Describe the auscultation of the chest, heart, and abdomen.**

Chest p. 81
Have your patient breathe more deeply and slowly than normal with an open mouth. Using the stethoscope's disk, auscultate each side of the chest from the apex to the base every 5 cm, listening at each location for one full breath.

Heart pp. 88–89
Using the diaphragm of the stethoscope, listen for heart sounds at the 2nd through 5th intercostal spaces at both sternal borders and at the point of maximum impulse (PMI). Repeat the process using the bell of the stethoscope to discern lower-pitched sounds.

Abdomen p. 94
Using the stethoscope's disk, auscultate each abdominal quadrant for at least 30 seconds to 1 minute.

12. **Distinguish between normal and abnormal auscultation findings of the chest, heart, and abdomen and explain their significance.**

Chest pp. 81–82
Normal breath sounds are the quiet sounds (almost low-pitched sighs) of air moving. Abnormal breath sounds are termed adventitious, and include the following. Any crackles (a light crackling, popping, non-musical sound) suggest fluid in the smaller airways. Late inspiratory crackles suggest heart failure or interstitial lung disease, while early crackles suggest heart failure or chronic bronchitis. Wheezes (more musical notes) denote obstruction of the smaller airways. The closer they appear to inspiration, the more serious the obstruction is. Stridor is a high-pitched, loud inspiratory wheeze reflective of laryngeal or tracheal obstruction. Grating or squeaking sounds describe pleural friction rubs and occur as the pleural layers become inflamed, then rub together. You may also listen for sound transmission while the patient speaks. Bronchophony occurs when you hear the words "ninety-nine" abnormally clearly through the stethoscope, a suggestion that blood, fluid, or a tumor has replaced normal tissue. Assess for whispered pectoriloquy by asking the patient to whisper "ninety-nine"; unusually clear sounds indicate an abnormal condition. Egophony occurs when you can hear the sound of long "e" as "a" when vocal resonance is abnormally increased.

Heart pp. 88–89
The normal heart produces a "lub-dub" sound heard through the disk of the stethoscope with each cardiac contraction. The "lub" and "dub" may split when valves close out of sync, "la-lub-dub" reflects an S_1 split while "lub-da-dub" is an S_2 split. S_2 splitting is normal in children and young adults, though abnormal in older adults if expiratory or persistent splitting occurs. S_3 splitting produces a "lub-dub-dee" cadence like the word "Kentucky." It occurs commonly in children and young adults, but reflects blood filling a dilated ventricle and may suggest ventricular

failure in the patient over 30. The S_4 heart sound is the "dee" sound of "dee-lub-dub" with a cadence similar to the word "Tennessee." It develops from vibrations as the atrium pushes blood into a ventricle that resists filling, suggestive of heart failure.

Abdomen   p. 94
Normal bowel sounds consist of a variety of high-pitched gurgles and clicks that occur every 5 to 15 seconds. More frequent activity suggests an increase in bowel motility and especially loud and prolonged gurgling sounds (borborygmi) indicate hyperperistalsis. Decreased or absent sounds suggest a paralytic ileus or peritonitis. You may also hear swishing sounds (bruit) over the major vessels suggesting vascular defect such as aneurysm or stenosis.

13. Describe special techniques of the cardiovascular examination.

Inspection for signs of cardiovascular insufficiency   p. 86
Examine the extremities for signs of insufficiency including pallor, delayed capillary refill, temperature variation, and dependent edema. Then assess the carotid arteries for pulse strength, rate, and rhythm. Does the rate or strength vary with respirations? Do you feel thrills (feel a humming sensation)? If so, auscultate for bruits.

Jugular vein distention   pp. 86, 88
Position the patient supine with the head elevated 30° and turned away from the side being assessed. Look for pulsations of the external jugular vein on either side of the trachea just before it passes behind the manubrium. Locate the highest point of pulsation and measure the distance from the sternal angle. Normal venous pressure distends the vein above the clavicle between 1 to 2 cm. Examine both jugulars for symmetrical pulsing and distention.

Point of maximum impulse (PMI)   p. 88
Have the patient lie comfortably with his head elevated 30°. Inspect and palpate the chest for the apical impulse or the PMI. It is normally at the 5th intercostal space, mid-clavicular line. In muscular or obese patients, you may need to percuss the point (dull vs. resonant).

CONTENT SELF-EVALUATION

MULTIPLE CHOICE

1. The layer of tissue that covers the interior of the chest wall and helps assure that the lungs move with the thorax is the:
   A. visceral pleura
   B. parietal pleura
   C. pertioneum
   D. pulmonary pleura
   E. perineum

2. A likely location to notice retraction during forced inspiration is:
   A. the suprasternal notch
   B. the intercostal spaces
   C. the supraclavicular space
   D. all of the above
   E. none of the above

3. The type of motion associated with a free segment of the chest where the segment moves opposite to the rest of the chest during breathing is:
   A. symbiotic
   B. paradoxical
   C. antagonistic
   D. retractive
   E. traumatic

4. During the palpation of the chest, you should feel for which of the following?
   A. tenderness
   B. deformities
   C. depressions
   D. asymmetry
   E. all of the above

_____ 5. During the check for chest excursion, the distance between your thumbs should increase by what amount during the patient's inspiration?
   A. 2 cm
   B. 3 to 5 cm
   C. 5 to 6 cm
   D. 10 to 12 cm
   E. the hands should not move

_____ 6. Increased tactile fremitus suggests which of the following conditions?
   A. pneumonia
   B. pneumothorax
   C. pleural effusion
   D. emphysema
   E. all of the above

_____ 7. Which condition is most likely to cause an area of the lung that is dull to percussion?
   A. pneumothorax
   B. tension pneumothorax
   C. hemothorax
   D. pericardial tamponade
   E. friction rubs

_____ 8. Light popping, nonmusical sounds heard in the chest during inspiration are known as:
   A. rhonchi
   B. stridor
   C. crackles
   D. wheezes
   E. none of the above

_____ 9. Hearing words transmitted clearly as you auscultate the chest with the stethoscope is a normal finding called bronchophony.
   A. True
   B. False

_____ 10. The point of maximal impulse (PMI) in the adult is usually located at the:
   A. 3rd costal cartilage, close to the sternum
   B. 3rd intercostal space, just left of the sternum
   C. 5th intercostal space, just right of the sternum
   D. 5th intercostal space, near the midclavicular line
   E. 8th intercostal space, near the midclavicular line

_____ 11. Which listing below represents the valves of the heart in order as blood flows through them from the vena cavae?
   A. tricuspid, pulmonic, mitral, aortic
   B. mitral, aortic, tricuspid, pulmonic
   C. pulmonic, tricuspid, aortic, mitral
   D. aortic, tricuspid, pulmonic, mitral
   E. tricuspid, aortic, mitral, pulmonic

_____ 12. The "lub" of the heart sounds represents which event of the cardiac cycle?
   A. ejection of blood from the ventricles
   B. ventricular contraction
   C. ventricular filling
   D. closing of the aortic and pulmonic valves
   E. closing of the tricuspid and mitral valves

_____ 13. Which of the following elements does NOT affect cardiac output?
   A. rate
   B. cardiac preload
   C. systolic blood pressure
   D. ventricular filling
   E. peripheral vascular resistance

_____ 14. Which of the following does NOT inhibit venous return to the heart?
   A. peripheral vascular resistance
   B. hypovolemia
   C. tension pneumothorax
   D. cardiac tamponade
   E. congestive heart failure

_____ 15. Which abdominal organ is found in all four quadrants?
   A. stomach
   B. liver
   C. large intestine
   D. pancreas
   E. spleen

_____ 16. An eccyhmotic discoloration over the umbilicus is:
A. Grey-Turner's sign
B. borborygami
C. Hering-Breuer sign
D. Cullen's sign
E. none of the above

_____ 17. Auscultation of high-pitched gurgles and clicks every 5 to 15 seconds in the abdomen indicates:
A. borborygmi
B. increased bowel motility
C. absent bowel sounds
D. normal bowel sounds
E. ascites

_____ 18. The fleshy folds that cover the vagina are the:
A. labia
B. clitoris
C. mons pubis
D. perineum
E. menarche

_____ 19. The sound or feeling caused by unlubricated bone ends rubbing together is:
A. palpable fremitus
B. crepitation
C. bruit
D. friction rub
E. the pooh-pooh sign

_____ 20. The type of movement permitted between the phalanges is:
A. abduction/adduction
B. rotation
C. flexion/extension
D. supination/pronation
E. both C and D

_____ 21. Carpal tunnel syndrome involves which nerve?
A. brachial
B. median
C. radial
D. ulnar
E. olecranon

_____ 22. The type of movement permitted between the radius, ulna, and humerus is:
A. abduction/adduction
B. rotation
C. flexion/extension
D. supination/pronation
E. both C and D

_____ 23. The joint which has the greatest range of motion of any joint in the human body is the:
A. shoulder
B. wrist
C. hip
D. elbow
E. ankle

_____ 24. A major muscle of the calf is the:
A. bicep
B. tricep
C. gastrocnemius
D. hamstring
E. gracilis anterior

_____ 25. The knee joint involves all of the following bones EXCEPT the:
A. femur
B. patella
C. tibia
D. fibula
E. all of the above

_____ 26. The type of motion permitted by the knee joint is:
A. flexion/extension
B. adduction/abduction
C. inversion/eversion
D. limited rotation
E. both A and D

_____ 27. Which region of the spine is most mobile?
A. cervical
B. thoracic
C. lumbar
D. sacral
E. coccygeal

_____ 28. The mid and lower cervical spine permits which type of movement?
    A. flexion   D. rotation
    B. extension   E. all of the above
    C. lateral bending

_____ 29. A lateral curvature of the spine is:
    A. lordosis
    B. scoliosis   D. spina bifida
    C. kyphosis   E. none of the above

_____ 30. Tenderness at a vertebral process and in the surrounding musculature of the lumbar spine is most likely due to:
    A. vertebral process fracture   D. herniated intervertebral disk
    B. ligamentous injury   E. none of the above
    C. paravertebral muscular spasm

SPECIAL PROJECTS

Range of Motion Exercise

Identify the range of motion for each of the joints listed in the chart below as discussed in your reading. Then fill in the rest by reviewing the text, pages 103 through 126.

It is not easy to remember and evaluate the range of motion for each joint of the extremities. To help you both remember the ranges of motion for each joint and assess the mobility of the patients you will treat, test your own joints for their range of motions against those from the text (and the chart below). Identify the joints where your movement exceeds or is less than the figures given in the book. Remember this difference. Then if you ever question how a patient's range of movements relates to the normal ranges, compare the patient's joint mobility to your own.

Upper Extremity

Joint	Flexion/Extension	Rotation	Other Motion
Wrist	_____/_____		(Medial/Lateral) _____/_____
Elbow	_____/_____		(Supination/Pronation) _____/_____
Shoulder	_____/_____	(Internal/External) _____/_____	(Abduction/Adduction) _____/_____

Lower Extremity

Joint	Flexion/Extension	Rotation	Other Motion
Ankle	(Dorsiflex/Plantar Flex) _____/_____		(Inversion/Eversion) _____/_____
Knee	_____/_____		
Hip	_____/_____	(External/Internal) _____/_____	(Abduction) _____

Physical Assessment—Personal Benchmarking

To perform the physical assessment of a patient, you will need to use the skills of inspection, palpation, auscultation, and percussion. You must not only master each of these skills but also learn to recognize normal and abnormal patient presentations. Often the distinction between normal and abnormal is very small and difficult to recognize without extensive experience. It is also difficult to maintain the ability to differentiate between normal and abnormal signs unless you practice the skill regularly. To help in skills maintenance, frequently use yourself as a physiologic model upon which to practice assessment techniques and as a benchmark against which you can measure your patients' responses.

Auscultation: You need a stethoscope for this exercise.

Take the diaphragm of the stethoscope and apply it to the skin of your chest or abdomen. If you do not warm it first, you will be quite surprised at how cold it feels. Remember this as you are auscultating your patients' chests and abdomens.

Practice using the disk and diaphragm to assure you know which setting sends bell sounds to your ears and which sends diaphragm sounds. Listen to the different sounds found at various locations around the chest and abdomen. Increase the pressure on the bell from gentle for low sounds to strong pressure for high-pitched sounds. You might also practice listening with the television on at various volume levels. This simulates background noise at the emergency scene and demonstrates how difficult it can be to assess breath, heart, and bowel sounds in the field.

Lung sounds: Review pages 81 through 83.

Listen to lung sounds in each of the five lung lobes. Remember that your patient's position will be reversed, his left lobes will be to your right. Take slow, deep breaths with your mouth open and listen for the faint noise of air moving through the small airways (normal or vesicular breath sounds). If you have a chance to auscultate your chest when you are experiencing the congestion of a cold, you may hear crackles or wheezes.

Then, auscultate the trachea at the suprasternal notch. Listen to the sounds, then move the diaphragm downward and laterally toward the lung fields. You will notice the quality of the sounds change as you move through the bronchial and bronchovesicular areas. Speak as you auscultate and notice how the speech sounds. It should be muffled, though you will hear it more clearly than when performing it on a patient because some sound is transmitted through the bones of the face and skull in addition to the stethoscope.

Heart sounds: Review pages 85 through 89.

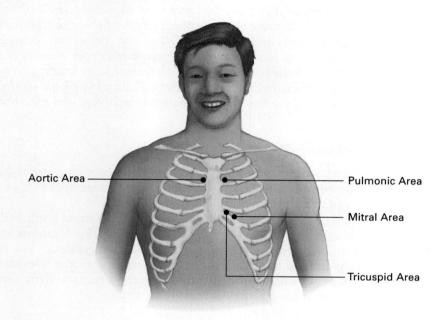

Aortic Area

Pulmonic Area

Mitral Area

Tricuspid Area

Review the accompanying illustration to identify the proper locations for auscultating the heart sounds. With each sound, increase the pressure on the bell from very light to heavy and appreciate the changing quality of the sounds. You might also palpate the carotid artery and then the radial pulse while auscultating to note the synchronization and delay between the sounds and pulse. Listen for the S_1 and S_2 sounds (the "lub-dub") of the normal heart.

Bowel sounds: Review page 94.

Review the text on page 94 and listen in each abdominal quadrant for at least 30 seconds to 1 minute with the diaphragm of your stethoscope. Listen very carefully in a very quiet environment, as bowel sounds are difficult to decipher. Check your bowel sounds at various times during the day. They will likely be most frequent just before and right after a meal and before you go to sleep.

CHAPTER 2
*
Physical Exam Techniques

Section III, pp. 128–165

Review of Chapter Objectives

After reading this chapter, you should be able to:

2. Describe the evaluation of mental status. pp. 134–137

The evaluation of the mental status begins with your interview. The evaluation permits you to determine your patient's level of responsiveness, general appearance, behavior, and speech. You specifically look at his appearance and behavior, speech and language skills, mood, thought and perception, insight and judgment, and memory and attention.

4. Describe the examination of the following body regions, differentiate between normal and abnormal findings, and define the significance of abnormal findings.

Peripheral vascular system pp. 128–133

Examine the upper, then the lower extremities and compare them, one to another, for the following: size, symmetry, swelling, venous congestion, skin and nail bed color, temperature, skin texture, and turgor. Yellow brittle nails, swollen digit ends (clubbing), or poor nailbed color suggest chronic arterial insufficiency. Assess the distal circulation, noting the strength, rate, and regularity of the pulse and comparing pulses bilaterally. If you have difficulty palpating a pulse or can't find one, palpate a more proximal site. Feel the spongy compliance of the vessels, note their coloration, and examine for inflammation along the vein, indicative of deep vein thrombosis. Gently feel for edema and pitting edema in each distal extremity.

Nervous system pp. 133–158

To evaluate mental status and speech, examine your patient's appearance and behavior, speech and language, mood, thoughts and perceptions, and memory and attention. Observe the patient's appearance and behavior, level of consciousness, posture and motor behavior, appropriateness of dress, grooming and personal hygiene, and the patient's facial expression. Note any abnormal speech pattern and observe the patient's attitude toward you and others expressed both verbally and non-verbally. Note any excessive emotion or lack of emotion. Assess the patient's thoughts and perceptions. Are they realistic and socially acceptable? Question for any visions, voices, perceived odors, or feelings about things that are not there. Examine the patient's insights and judgments to determine if he knows what is happening. Assess the patient's memory and attention and determine his orientation to time, place, and person (sometimes considered as person and own person). Then test immediate, recent, and remote memory. Any deviation from a normal and expected response is to be noted and suggests illness or psychiatric problem.

   Begin the examination of the motor system by observing the patient for symmetry, deformities, and involuntary movements. Tremors or fasiculations while the patient is at rest suggest

Parkinson's disease, while their occurrence during motion suggests postural tremor. Determine muscle bulk, which is classified as normal, atrophy, hypertrophy, or pseudotrophy (bulk without strength as in muscular dystrophy). Unilateral hand atrophy suggests median or ulnar nerve paralysis. Check tone by moving a relaxed limb through a range of motion. Describe any flaccidity or rigidity and then examine muscle strength starting with grip strength and continuing through all limbs. Again note any asymmetry (the patient's dominant side should be slightly stronger). Observe the patient's gait and have him walk a straight line (heel to toe). Any ataxia suggests cerebellar disease, loss of position sense, or intoxication. Also have the patient walk on his toes, then heels, hop on each foot, and then do a shallow knee bend. Perform a Romberg test (have him stand with his feet together and eyes closed for 20 to 30 seconds). Any excessive sway (a positive Romberg test) suggests ataxia from loss of position sense, while inability to maintain balance with eyes open represents cerebellar ataxia. Ask the patient to hold his arms straight out in front with his palms up and eyes closed. Pronation suggests mild hemiparesis, drifting sideways or upward suggests loss of positional sense. Ask your patient to perform various rapid alternating movements and observe for smoothness, speed, and rhythm. The dominant side should perform best, and any slow, irregular or clumsy movements suggest cerebellar or extrapyramidal disease. Have your patient touch his thumb rapidly with the tip of the index finger, place his hand on his thigh and rapidly alternate from palm up to down, and assess for point-to-point testing (touch his nose, then your index finger several times rapidly, or, for the legs, have him touch heel to knee, then run it down the shin). Any jerking, difficulty in performing the task, or tremors suggest cerebellar disease. For position testing, have the patient perform the leg test with his eyes closed.

Evaluate the sensory system by testing sensations of pain, light touch, temperature, position, vibration, and discrimination. Compare responses bilaterally and from distal to proximal, then associate any deficit discovered with the dermatome it represents. Test superficial and deep tendon reflexes and note a dulled (cord or lower neuron damage) or hyperactive response (upper neuron disease).

Cranial nerves pp. 137–147

CN-I is checked by evaluating the ability to sense odors in each nostril.

CN-II is checked by testing for visual acuity and field of view.

CN-III is checked by examining pupillary direct and consensual response.

CN-III, IV, and VI are checked by testing for smooth and unrestricted extraocular motion.

CN-V is checked by testing the masseter muscle strength and sensation on the forehead, cheek, chin, and cornea.

CN-VII is checked by examining the patient's face during conversations, looking for any asymmetry, eyelid droop, or abnormal movements.

CN-VIII is checked by evaluating for hearing and balance (with his eyes closed).

CN-IX and X are checked by evaluating speech, swallowing, saying "aaahhh," and the gag reflex.

CN-XI is checked by testing trapezius and sternocleidomastoid muscles at rest and by evaluating head turning and shoulder raising.

CN-XII is checked by evaluating speech and having the patient extend his tongue outward.

Any deviation from a normally expected response is a reason to suspect a cranial nerve injury.

14. Describe the general guidelines of recording examination information. pp. 164–168

Use a standard format to organize the information. Use appropriate medical terminology and language. Present your findings legibly, accurately, and truthfully, remembering that your record will become a legal document. Include all data discovered in your assessment.

The standard organization for medical documentation is the S (Subjective), O (Objective), A (Assessment), and P (Plan) format (SOAP format):

Subjective information is what your patient or others tell you, including the chief complaint and the past and present medical history.

Objective information is that which you observe or determine during the scene size-up, initial assessment, focused history and physical exam, detailed assessment, and ongoing assessments.

Assessment summarizes the findings to suggest a field diagnosis.

Plan is the further diagnosis, treatment, and patient education you intend to offer.

15. Discuss the examination considerations for an infant or child.   pp. 158–164

Children are not small adults, but patients with special physiological and psychological differences. In general, remain calm and confident, establish a rapport with the parents, and have them help with the exam. Provide positive feedback to both the child and parents.

The transition from newborn to adulthood is a continuum of development, both physically and emotionally. When assessing pediatric patients, keep the following differences from adults in mind:

The bones of the skull do not close until about 18 months and joints remain cartilaginous until 5 years.

The child's airway is narrow and will be more quickly and severely obstructed than the adult's.

Instead of listening for verbal complaints, note the child's eyes, expression, and the degree of activity it takes to distract him from the problem as an indication of its seriousness.

Rib fractures are rare due to the cartilaginous nature of the ribs, though the tissue underneath is more prone to injury.

The liver and spleen are proportionally large and are more subject to injury.

Children are more likely to experience bone injury rather than ligament and tendon injury.

Normal vital signs for children will change through the stages of their development.

CONTENT SELF-EVALUATION

MULTIPLE CHOICE

_____ 1. A normal pulse quality would be reported as:
   A. 0   D. 3+
   B. 1+   E. 4+
   C. 2+

_____ 2. Which of the following is NOT a sign of proximal arterial occlusion?
   A. thrills   D. poor color in the fingertips
   B. pulse deficit   E. slow capillary refill
   C. cold limb

_____ 3. Pitting edema that depresses 1/2 to 1 inch is reported as:
   A. 0   D. 3+
   B. 1+   E. 4+
   C. 2+

_____ 4. The pitting of edema will usually disappear within how many seconds after the release of pressure?
   A. 2   D. 8
   B. 4   E. 10
   C. 6

_____ 5. A complete neurological exam includes which of the following areas?
   A. cranial nerves   D. sensory system
   B. motor system   E. all of the above
   C. reflexes

_____ 6. The cerebral cortex is the center for which of the following?
   A. conscious thought   D. emotions
   B. sensory awareness   E. all of the above
   C. movement

_____ 7. A patient who is drowsy but answers questions is considered to be:
   A. lethargic   D. comatose
   B. obtunded   E. none of the above
   C. stuporous

_____ 8. Normal speech is:
  A. inflected
  B. clear and strong
  C. fluent and articulate
  D. varies in volume
  E. all of the above

_____ 9. The term dysphonia refers to which of the following?
  A. defective speech caused by motor deficits
  B. voice changes due to vocal cord problems
  C. defective language due to neurologic problem
  D. voice changes due to aging
  E. none of the above

_____ 10. The term aphasia refers to which of the following?
  A. defective speech caused by motor deficits
  B. voice changes due to vocal cord problems
  C. defective language due to a neurologic problem
  D. voice changes due to aging
  E. none of the above

_____ 11. Which of the following is one of the three basic grades of memory:
  A. intermediate
  B. verifiable
  C. redux
  D. remote
  E. retrograde

_____ 12. A question about a patient's wife's birthday tests which of the following types of memory?
  A. intermediate
  B. verifiable
  C. redux
  D. remote
  E. retrograde

_____ 13. During the test of extraoccular eye movement you should trace which figure in front of your patient's eyes?
  A. an "X"
  B. an "H"
  C. a "+"
  D. a large "O"
  E. any of the above

_____ 14. Stimulation for a blink by touching the eye's surface with fine cotton fibers tests which of the following?
  A. corneal reflex
  B. ptosis
  C. EOM
  D. the trigeminal nerve
  E. none of the above

_____ 15. When a person loses his sense of balance, which cranial nerve has most likely been injured?
  A. equilibrial
  B. glossopharyngeal
  C. acoustic
  D. vagus
  E. accessory

_____ 16. Damage to CN-12 will cause the tongue to deviate in which manner?
  A. downward
  B. upward
  C. toward the side of injury
  D. away from the side of injury
  E. furrow and curve upward

_____ 17. The pyramidal pathway within the spinal cord mediates which of the following?
  A. voluntary muscle control
  B. involuntary muscle control
  C. dermatome sensation
  D. visceral sensation
  E. vasoconstriction

_____ 18. Damage to the extrapyramidal pathways is likely to cause what type of presentation?
  A. abnormal posture
  B. abnormal gait
  C. involuntary movement
  D. increased muscle tone
  E. all of the above

_____ 19. The twitching of small muscle fibers is:
  A. spasm
  B. tics
  C. tremors
  D. fasciculations
  E. atrophy

_____ 20. In cases of muscular dystrophy, the patient's muscles:
  A. increase in size
  B. decrease in size
  C. increase in strength
  D. decrease in strength
  E. both A and D

_____ 21. During your testing of a patient's muscle strength, you notice one side to be slightly stronger than the other. This is a normal finding.
  A. True
  B. False

_____ 22. Which of the following procedures describes the Romberg test? Have the patient:
  A. walk heel-to-toe in a straight line
  B. stand with eyes closed for 20 to 30 seconds
  C. walk across the room and turn and walk back again
  D. do a shallow knee bend on each leg in turn
  E. walk first on his heels, then toes

_____ 23. An area of skin innervated by a specific peripheral nerve root is a(n):
  A. afferent region
  B. sensory topographic region
  C. myotome
  D. dermatome
  E. both A and C

_____ 24. The score on the muscle strength scale that describes a patient able to perform active movement against gravity is:
  A. 5
  B. 4
  C. 3
  D. 2
  E. 1

_____ 25. Babinski's response is positive when the sole of the foot is stroked and:
  A. the big toe plantar flexes while other toes dorsiflex
  B. the big toe plantar flexes while other toes fan out
  C. the big toe dorsiflexes while other toes fan out
  D. the big toe dorsiflexes while other toes plantar flex
  E. all toes plantar flex

_____ 26. In caring for the ill or injured child, it is important to be which of the following?
  A. confident
  B. direct
  C. honest
  D. calm
  E. all of the above

_____ 27. Children first recognize their parents' faces and voices at about what age?
  A. 2 months
  B. 6 months
  C. 8 months
  D. 10 months
  E. 1 year

_____ 28. Infants begin to sit up at about what age?
  A. 2 to 4 months
  B. 4 to 6 months
  C. 6 to 8 months
  D. 10 months to 1 year
  E. 1 year or later

_____ 29. The most difficult pediatric age group to assess is the:
  A. infant   D. school age
  B. toddler   E. adolescent
  C. preschooler

_____ 30. Which of the following groups is particularly distrusting of strangers?
  A. infant   D. school age
  B. toddler   E. adolescent
  C. preschooler

_____ 31. The soft spots in the skull, called fontanelles, close at about what age?
  A. 6 months   D. 24 months
  B. 12 months   E. 30 months
  C. 18 months

_____ 32. Bulging along the sutures of the skull of a young child suggests which of the following?
  A. dehydration
  B. reduced venous pressure in the jugular veins
  C. decreased arterial pressure
  D. arterial blockage to the cerebrum
  E. none of the above

_____ 33. Because the tissue of the child's upper airway is so flexible, injuries, infections, or minor obstructions do not adversely affect it as seriously as they would an adult's.
  A. True
  B. False

_____ 34. Which of the following statements regarding the chest of an infant or small child is FALSE?
  A. Children have a less mobile mediastinum than adults.
  B. The chest is rather elastic.
  C. The chest is rather flexible.
  D. Chest fractures are less likely.
  E. The chest is comprised of more cartilage than the adult's.

_____ 35. Because of the structure of the thoracic cage, the child is less likely to develop tension pneumothorax than the adult.
  A. True
  B. False

_____ 36. The normal respiratory rate for an infant is:
  A. 30 to 50 breaths per minute   D. 22 to 34 breaths per minute
  B. 30 to 60 breaths per minute   E. 18 to 30 breaths per minute
  C. 24 to 40 breaths per minute

_____ 37. The normal systolic blood pressure for the newborn is:
  A. 60 to 90   D. 95 to 110
  B. 87 to 105   E. 112 to 128
  C. 95 to 105

_____ 38. Which of the following is NOT true regarding the abdomen of the child?
  A. The liver is proportionally larger than the adult's.
  B. The spleen is proportionally larger than the adult's.
  C. The abdominal muscles provide less protection than the adult's.
  D. The abdomen rarely bulges at the end of inspiration.
  E. Inguinal hernias are common in young children.

_____ 39. Which of the following statements is true regarding the recording of examination findings?
   A. The patient care report is only as good as the accuracy, detail, and depth you provide.
   B. The patient chart is a legal document.
   C. The absence of an expected sign in a patient may be just as important as its presence.
   D. The universally accepted organization for recording patient information is SOAP.
   E. all of the above

_____ 40. The patient's chief complaint is recorded under which element of the SOAP documentation format?
   A. S
   B. O
   C. A
   D. P
   E. none of the above

MATCHING

Match the cranial nerve number with its name and function by writing the appropriate numbers in the spaces provided.

Cranial Nerve	Name	Function
41. I	_____	_____
42. II	_____	_____
43. III	_____	_____
44. IV	_____	_____
45. V	_____	_____
46. VI	_____	_____
47. VII	_____	_____
48. VIII	_____	_____
49. IX	_____	_____
50. X	_____	_____
51. XI	_____	_____
52. XII	_____	_____

Name
   a. Acoustic
   b. Optic
   c. Trochlear
   d. Abducens
   e. Accessory
   f. Glossopharyngeal
   g. Trigeminal
   h. Oculomotor
   i. Vagus
   j. Hypoglossal
   k. Facial
   l. Olfactory

Function
   m. Smell
   n. Posterior palate and pharynx motor control
   o. Trapezius and sternocleidomastoid motor control
   p. Sight
   q. Tongue sensation
   r. Motor control of the tongue
   s. Motor control of the superior oblique muscles
   t. Anterior tongue sensation posterior pharynx motor control
   u. Lateral rectus muscle motor control
   v. Hearing and balance
   w. Eye movement and pupil constriction
   x. Forehead, cheek, and chin sensation

SPECIAL PROJECTS

Physical Assessment—Personal Benchmarking

To perform the physical assessment of a patient, you will need to use the skills of inspection, palpation, auscultation, and percussion. You must not only master each of these skills but also learn to recognize normal and abnormal patient presentations. Often the distinction between normal and abnormal is very small and difficult to recognize without extensive experience. It is also difficult to maintain the ability to differentiate between normal and abnormal signs unless you practice the skill regularly. To help in skills maintenance, use yourself as a physiologic model upon which to practice assessment techniques and as a benchmark against which you can measure your patients' responses.

Pulse location and evaluation: Review pages 128 and 130 through 132.

Palpate each of the following arteries for the location, rate, and strength of pulsation.

> Radial—wrist, thumb side
> Ulnar—wrist, little finger side
> Brachial—medial aspect, just above the elbow
> Carotid—just lateral of the trachea (palpate both)
> Femoral—half the distance between the anterior iliac crest (the bone the belt sits on) and the
>   symphysis pubis (just below the inguinal ligament)
> Popliteal—just behind and below the knee
> Posterior tibial—below the medial malleolus (ankle bone)
> Dorsalis pedis—on top of the foot

Locate each of these pulses on yourself, but realize that you are healthy and perfusing well. It is more difficult to find and evaluate these distal pulses on patients, especially the pulses on the lower extremities and those of patients with serious medical or trauma-induced problems. Remember to place the pads of your fingers lightly over the artery and increase the pressure until you feel the strongest impulse. Rate each pulse from 0 to 3+ (with 0 = absent, 1+ = weak or thready, 2+ = normal, 3+ = bounding). Practice finding and rating the pulses quickly. These skills will be invaluable when you go to assess your patients.

You might try counting a pulse in your arm or forearm while driving or riding in a car. The vibration of travel makes the task much harder and simulates pulse evaluation in a moving ambulance. It might also be helpful to assess the pulses of friends and fellow emergency care workers to gain invaluable practice.

Ausculation Exercise

Indicate the proper locations at which to auscultate heart sounds on the accompanying illustration. Be sure to include locations for auscultation of sounds in the aortic, pulmonic, mitral, and tricuspid areas as well as the point of maximal impulse.

CHAPTER 3

*

Patient Assessment in the Field

Because Chapter 3 is lengthy, it has been divided into sections to aid your study. Read the assigned text pages, then progress through the objectives and self-evaluation materials as you would with other chapters. When you feel secure in your grasp of the content, proceed to the next section.

Section I, pp. 170–200

Review of Chapter Objectives

After reading this chapter, you should be able to:

1. Recognize hazards/potential hazards associated with the medical and trauma scene.   **pp. 174–182**

During the scene size-up, you must examine the scene before you arrive at the patient's side. It is a time to evaluate and prepare for hazards including blood, fluids, airborne pathogens, and other conditions that may threaten your life or health. These conditions include the hazards of fire, structural collapse, traffic, unstable surfaces, electricity, broken glass, or jagged metal. Hazardous materials can involve chemical spills, radiation, and toxic environments. Finally, scene hazards can also include violent, disturbed, or unruly bystanders or patients. These hazards are not limited to the trauma scene but may be found at many medical scenes as well.

2. Identify unsafe scenes and describe methods for making them safe.   **pp. 174–182**

Your responsibility at the emergency scene is to recognize hazards including fire, structural collapse, traffic, unstable surfaces, electricity, broken glass, jagged metal, and hazardous materials and then act appropriately to protect yourself, other rescuers, and your patient. Unless you are specially trained and equipped to handle a specific hazard, do not enter the scene. In most cases, you will rely on the fire department, rescue service, police department, power company, hazmat team, or other specially trained personnel to secure the scene before you enter. If there is ever a question of whether a scene is safe or unsafe, do not enter the scene.

3. Discuss common mechanisms of injury/nature of illness.   **pp. 184–185**

Trauma is induced by a mechanism of injury through which forces enter the body and do physical harm. Common mechanisms include blunt trauma—for example, vehicle crashes (auto, recreational, watercraft, and bicycle), pedestrian vs. vehicle impacts, falls—and penetrating trauma—for example, gunshot and knife wounds. Medical problems have a related cause called the nature of the illness. The scene can provide evidence as to the nature of the illness. Examples include the presence of nebulizers, which suggest asthma, drug paraphernalia, which suggest overdose, and medications, which suggest preexisting cardiac or other problems.

4. Predict patterns of injury based on mechanism of injury. pp. 184–185, 200–201

Analyze the strength, direction, and nature of the forces expressed to the patient during the incident. This analysis will suggest the probable type of injury, the organs involved, and the seriousness of injury. In a vehicle crash, for example, such things as a broken windshield, a bent steering wheel, an intrusion into the passenger compartment, and the use of restraints by occupants can suggest potential injuries and their severity. Types of injuries can also be predicted for each type of vehicle crash—frontal, lateral, rear-end, rotational, and rollover. The analysis of the accident can lead to your anticipation of possible injuries, or an index of suspicion.

5. Discuss the reason for identifying the total number of patients at the scene. pp. 182–183

Determining the number of patients at a scene is important to assure that the needed resources are summoned to the scene and that every patient is cared for. At each and every scene, you should ask yourself, "Could there be others who are injured or ill?" While at the trauma scene it is common to find a patient wandering among the bystanders, the medical scene can have "hidden patients" too. The wife of a cardiac arrest patient, for example, may herself become a patient because of the emotional stress of the incident. Knowing the number of patients can help you gauge whether on-scene resources are adequate or whether you need to request that additional units and manpower be dispatched to the scene. The earlier this request is made, the quicker those resources will arrive.

6. Organize the management of a scene following size-up. pp. 185–200

The management of the scene following the scene size-up includes requesting both the appropriate units and personnel to manage scene hazards and the appropriate number and care levels of ambulances and personnel to treat the patients. You must also take the necessary steps to assure overall scene safety and to protect yourself, the patient, other scene personnel, and bystanders. The scene size-up also prepares you to manage the care of the patient by helping you recognize the mechanism of injury and anticipate injuries (index of suspicion) or by recognizing the nature of the illness.

7. Explain the reasons for identifying the need for additional help or assistance during the scene size-up. pp. 176–183

Multiple patients at the emergency scene can rapidly overwhelm your ability to provide effective care. If you wait until you are at a patient's side before calling for additional help, you may be distracted from making the call and delay an effective response. In cases where the number of patients far outstrips your ability to provide care, you may need to initiate a mass casualty response.

8. Summarize the reasons for forming a general impression of the patient. pp. 186–187

The initial general impression of your patient takes into account the patient's age, gender, race, and other factors that will help you determine the seriousness of the problem and establish your priorities for patient care and transport. As you learn more about the patient through the initial assessment and the focused history and physical assessment, you will refine and improve on the accuracy and depth of the general impression. As you develop your general impression of the patient early in the assessment process, you can also begin to establish a rapport with him or her, explaining why you are there, what will be happening to him or her, and giving the patient the opportunity to refuse care.

9. Discuss methods of assessing mental status/levels of consciousness in the adult, infant, and child patient. pp. 187–189

Initially determine the patient's mental status by categorizing him according to the AVPU system. Using this method, the patient is classified either Alert, responsive to Verbal stimuli, responsive to Painful stimuli, or Unresponsive. You can further refine the evaluation by questioning the patient to determine orientation to place, time, and person and by differentiating his or her response to pain into purposeful and purposeless movement and decerebrate and decorticate posturing. An alert response for the infant or child is difficult to assess because of that patient's limited speech capabilities. Evaluate pediatric patients for activity and curiosity, being aware that the quiet child is often a seriously ill or injured one.

10. Discuss methods of assessing and securing the airway in the adult, child, and infant patient. pp. 189–195

The patient who is speaking clearly (or the child or infant who is crying loudly) has a patent airway. For other patients, position your head at the patient's mouth and look, listen, and feel for air moving through the airway. If you detect no movement, open the airway by using either the jaw thrust (in patients with trauma and suspected spine injury) or the head-tilt/chin-lift. Suction any fluids from the airway and remove obstructions using the Heimlich maneuver or laryngoscopy with Magill forceps. Secure the airway, as needed, with an oral or nasal airway, endotracheal intubation, or creation of a needle or surgical airway. When you have a pediatric patient, be sure to position the head and neck properly (using slight extension and padding under the shoulders), taking account of the differences in the pediatric anatomy. Also, reduce the size of the airways, laryngoscope blades, and endotracheal tubes you use with these patients.

11. State reasons for cervical spine management for the trauma patient. p. 187

The spinal cord is the major communication distribution and collection conduit for the central nervous system. It is protected by the spinal column, the bony and flexible structure that runs from the base of the skull to just below the pelvis. If the column is injured, it may become unstable and permit injury to the spinal cord. Because injuries to the cord have such serious consequences, you should immobilize the spine early in your assessment and care to protect this essential communication pathway. Its immobilization will not harm the patient, while uncontrolled movement can cause permanent spinal cord injury.

12. Analyze a scene to determine if spinal precautions are required. pp. 184–185, 200–202

Your examination of the scene and the analysis of the mechanism of injury will suggest or rule out the potential for spinal injury. The patient with a significant mechanism of injury—severe vehicle crash, fall from a height, injury causing a major long bone fracture, or any injury or mechanism of injury that suggests the body was subjected to significant trauma forces—has a likelihood of spinal fracture and requires spinal precautions.

13. Describe methods for assessing respiration in the adult, child, and infant patient. pp. 194–195

If your patient is speaking clearly (or if an infant or child patient is crying loudly) presume the airway is clear. Otherwise, listen for the sounds of airway restriction or obstruction, such as gurgling, stridor, or wheezes. If airway sounds are absent, place your ear at the patient's mouth while you listen, watch, and feel for air movement through it. If there is any doubt about airway patency, position the head with the jaw thrust or head-tilt/chin-lift. With a child, do not hyperextend the neck as this may block the airway. You may have to place padding behind the shoulders of a small child or infant to maintain proper head positioning.

14. Describe the methods used to locate and assess a pulse in the adult, child, and infant patient. pp. 195–196

Use the pads of your fingers and apply gentle, increasing pressure until you feel a strong pulsing over the radial artery in the adult and brachial artery in the small child or infant. If the radial or brachial pulse cannot be felt, check the carotid or, in the infant, the apical pulse. An adult radial pulse generally suggests a blood pressure of at least 80 mmHg, while a carotid pulse suggests a systolic blood pressure of at least 60 mmHg. Pulse rates usually decrease with age from a high of 100 to 180 in the infant to 60 to 100 in the adult. The pulse should be strong and regular.

15. **Discuss the need for assessing the patient for external bleeding.**   pp. 195–198

The patient with the potential for external hemorrhage must be assessed to determine both the nature and the extent of the blood loss. Any significant external hemorrhage must be halted and the amount of loss approximated to help prevent hypovolemia and to determine what effects the loss will have on the patient's body.

16. **Describe normal and abnormal findings when assessing skin color, temperature, and condition.**   p. 198

Normal skin is warm, moist, and pink in color (in light-skinned people), reflecting good perfusion. The body's compensation for shock results in vasoconstriction, which produces mottled, cyanotic, pale or ashen skin color, and skin that is cool to the touch. Capillary refill times may exceed 3 seconds, though this may be due to a number of preexisting conditions in adults.

17. **Explain the reason and process for prioritizing a patient for care and transport.**   pp. 198–200

At the conclusion of the initial assessment, you must determine your patient's priority, which will indicate how to proceed with assessment, care, and transport. With a seriously ill or injured patient, perform a rapid head-to-toe assessment. With a stable medical or trauma patient, perform a focused history and physical exam. You will also need to determine the priority for transport—either immediate transport with care rendered en route or with most care provided at the scene followed by transport.

18. **Use the findings of the initial assessment to determine the patient's perfusion status.**   p. 199

The initial assessment provides you with a general impression of the patient, a determination of the patient's mental status, and an evaluation of the airway, breathing, and circulation. This information indicates the status of the patient's respiration/oxygenation and circulation. It also indicates the patient's level of consciousness and the perfusion of the body's most important end-organ, the brain.

CASE STUDY REVIEW

Reread the case study on pages 172 and 173 in Paramedic Care: Patient Assessment *before reading the discussion below.*

This case study gives you the opportunity quickly to identify and review the elements of the patient assessment process. The process involves the scene size-up, initial assessment, focused history and physical exam, detailed exam, and ongoing assessments.

Even before Chris arrives at the scene, she uses the time available to her to review the elements of the scene size-up and her expected assessment and care. She identifies the likely mechanism of injury as a fall from a great height with an impact on an unforgiving surface. She suspects very serious injuries and the need for rapid assessment and care. Given the expected mechanism of injury, Chris may alert the trauma center to let them know of the incident and, if she is more than 15 minutes away from the center, might also put the helicopter service on standby.

As Chris arrives, she sizes up the scene and quickly determines that the dispatch information was correct. She dons her gloves to protect against the dangers of body substance contamination and requests additional help from the fire department. She also recognizes that this is not likely to be a hazardous scene but that she may have to contend with curious onlookers and those who are made emotionally distraught by the sight of blood and gore. Finally, Chris considers the mechanism of injury to help her anticipate injuries. Given the circumstances, Chris expects numerous broken bones, internal injuries, and head and spine trauma in this patient.

As Chris moves to the patient's side, she begins the initial assessment. She already has a general impression of the patient's condition, and it is not good. She builds upon this impression as the assessment continues. She immediately directs Nick to hold cervical spine stabilization as one of the first steps in the initial assessment. He continues manual stabilization until the patient is fully immobilized by mechanical means later on. Chris determines the patient is completely unresponsive and then moves to assess the ABCs. The airway is cleared, respirations are supported, and Chris begins treating the patient for shock. These actions are essential to sustain life, and Chris does not delay her initial assessment to care for any non-life-threatening injuries.

With the airway, breathing, and circulation stabilized, Chris moves to the rapid trauma assessment, a form of the focused history and physical exam. Here she concentrates her patient evaluation on possible critical injuries. She examines the head, neck, chest, abdomen, pelvis, and extremities and notes the depressed skull fracture, the rigid abdomen, and the pelvic and femur fractures. She also notes pertinent negatives (expected but not substantiated findings) like the absent signs of pneumothorax. Since this is a critical trauma patient, transport and life-sustaining interventions are the highest priorities, and Chris does not perform a detailed physical exam. Doing so would extend the time at the scene and probably not suggest any care steps that Chris and Nick are not already planning. The care team determines that their patient is critical and needs the services of a trauma center. They make arrangements to expedite transport.

Once the patient is on the way to the trauma center and all critical interventions have been performed, Chris provides an ongoing assessment. She quickly reevaluates the level of responsiveness, ABCs, vital signs, and the patient's signs and symptoms. She documents the results to track the patient's progress during her care—Is the patient improving, deteriorating, or remaining the same? Since the patient is critical, Chris performs the ongoing assessment every 5 minutes. (She would perform it every 15 minutes or so for a nonserious patient.) She also employs the ongoing assessment whenever her team performs an invasive procedure or anytime they notice a change in a patient sign or symptom.

CONTENT SELF-EVALUATION

MULTIPLE CHOICE

_____ 1. As a paramedic, you will certainly never perform a comprehensive history and physical exam in the acute setting.
    A. True
    B. False

_____ 2. Which component of the patient assessment process will be performed during patient transport?
    A. scene survey
    B. initial assessment
    C. focused history and physical exam
    D. detailed physical exam
    E. ongoing assessment

_____ 3. After the scene size-up and if necessary, you should inform the dispatcher of:
    A. the nature of the medical or trauma emergency
    B. what resources you need
    C. the phone number at which you can be reached
    D. what actions you and your crew are taking
    E. all of the above except C

_____ 4. Which of the following is NOT a component of the scene size-up?
    A. body substance isolation
    B. general impression of the patient
    C. location of all patients
    D. mechanism of injury/nature of the illness analysis
    E. scene safety

_____ 5. Which of the following body substance isolation devices will you employ with every patient you treat?
    A. latex or vinyl gloves   D. gown
    B. protective eyewear   E. both B and C
    C. face mask

_____ 6. Whenever you plan to intubate a patient, you should wear:
   A. latex or vinyl gloves and a gown
   B. protective eyewear, a gown, and a face mask
   C. latex or vinyl gloves, protective eyewear, and a face mask
   D. protective eyewear and a gown
   E. latex or vinyl gloves

_____ 7. The HEPA respirator is designed to filter out which of the following pathogens that may be encountered when providing prehospital emergency care?
   A. tuberculosis   D. the flu
   B. small pox   E. tetanus toxoid
   C. anthrax

_____ 8. The intent of the safety analysis portion of the scene survey is to assure the safety of:
   A. the patient   D. yourself
   B. bystanders   E. all of the above
   C. fellow responders

_____ 9. To properly handle a scene safety issue, you must be:
   A. properly trained
   B. properly equipped
   C. properly clothed
   D. prepared to attempt rescue procedures in which you have not been trained
   E. A, B, and C above

_____ 10. Potential hazards to rule out before entering the scene include all of the following EXCEPT:
   A. fire   D. structural collapse
   B. electrocution   E. broken glass and jagged metal
   C. contamination with blood

_____ 11. When called to a shooting or domestic disturbance, until the police arrive and secure the scene you should remain:
   A. outside the neighborhood   D. at the door but don't enter
   B. outside the residence   E. either B or C
   C. just down the street

_____ 12. At which of the following incidents would you NOT expect to discover more than one patient in your scene size-up?
   A. a two-car accident
   B. a carbon monoxide poisoning in a home
   C. a car crash in which a child seat and diaper bag are visible
   D. a fall out of a tree
   E. a hazardous materials spill in a high-school chemistry lab

_____ 13. You should delay the call for additional ambulances until you begin your initial assessment because you will not have enough information to determine the needs of the scene until then.
   A. True
   B. False

_____ 14. The two important functions that must begin immediately in the mass casualty situation are:
   A. triage and incident command   D. incident command and extrication
   B. rescue and triage   E. incident command and scene isolation
   C. fire fighting and rescue

_____ 15. The responsibilities of incident command at a disaster scene include all of the following EXCEPT:
   A. performing a scene size-up
   B. triaging initial patients for care
   C. determining the need for additional resources
   D. radioing for additional equipment and personnel
   E. directing in-coming crews

_____ 16. The responsibilities of the triage person at the disaster scene include all of the following EXCEPT:
   A. determining a patient's priority for immediate transport
   B. determining a patient's priority for delayed transport
   C. performing simple, but life-saving procedures
   D. providing intensive care on salvageable patients
   E. all of the above

_____ 17. The mechanism of injury analysis examines:
   A. body locations affected   D. nature of the crash forces
   B. strength of the crash forces   E. all of the above
   C. direction of the crash forces

_____ 18. The index of suspicion is best defined as:
   A. patient priority for care based on the MOI
   B. anticipation of the nature of forces involved in an accident
   C. anticipation of injuries based upon the MOI
   D. anticipation of degree of injury based on the patient's appearance
   E. none of the above

_____ 19. The nature of the illness is determined from information you receive from:
   A. the patient   D. scene clues
   B. the patient's family   E. all of the above
   C. bystanders

_____ 20. The initial assessment includes all of the following EXCEPT:
   A. forming a general impression of the patient
   B. stabilizing the cervical spine as needed
   C. immobilizing of fractures
   D. assessing the airway
   E. assessing the circulation

_____ 21. The general patient impression is based upon all of the following EXCEPT:
   A. blood pressure   D. the environment
   B. mechanism of injury   E. your instincts
   C. chief complaint

_____ 22. Which of the following is NOT a purpose served by your initial introduction to the patient?
   A. identifying yourself
   B. identifying your reason for being there
   C. establishing your level of training
   D. giving the patient an opportunity to refuse care
   E. establishing informed consent

_____ 23. During the initial assessment, the cervical spine should be stabilized:
   A. after the airway is established
   B. just before you attempt artificial ventilation
   C. immediately, if suggested by the MOI
   D. after the circulation check
   E. as the last step of the initial assessment

_____ 24. Which of the following conditions does NOT normally cause an altered mental status?
   A. eupnea
   B. drug overdose
   C. head injury
   D. poisoning
   E. sepsis

_____ 25. A patient who only moves his arm when firmly pinched between the thumb and first finger and shows no other responses will be classified as which of the following under the AVPU system?
   A. A
   B. V
   C. P
   D. U
   E. cannot be determined with the information at hand

_____ 26. A patient who is disoriented and confused would be classified as which of the following under the AVPU system?
   A. A
   B. V
   C. P
   D. U
   E. cannot be determined with the information at hand

_____ 27. Stridor can usually be caused by all of the following EXCEPT:
   A. infection
   B. gastric distress
   C. foreign body
   D. severe swelling
   E. allergic reaction

_____ 28. For stridor that is caused by respiratory burns, the care procedure most likely to maintain the airway is:
   A. suctioning
   B. blow-by oxygen and a quiet ride to the hospital
   C. a surgical airway
   D. early endotracheal intubation
   E. vasoconstrictor medications

_____ 29. A patient with abnormally deep respirations is said to be:
   A. hyperpneic
   B. tachypneic
   C. eupneic
   D. bradypneic
   E. hypopneic

_____ 30. The presence of a radial pulse suggests that the systolic blood pressure is at least:
   A. 60 mmHg
   B. 70 mmHg
   C. 80 mmHg
   D. 100 mmHg
   E. 120 mmHg

LISTING

List the components of patient assessment in the order they would be performed in the field.

31. _____

32. _____

33. _____

34. _____

35. _____

SPECIAL PROJECT

Scene Size-Up Exercise

Review the photographs below and identify the likely hazards you should suspect at each scene.

A. _____

_____

_____

_____

_____

_____

_____

_____

_____

_____

_____

_____

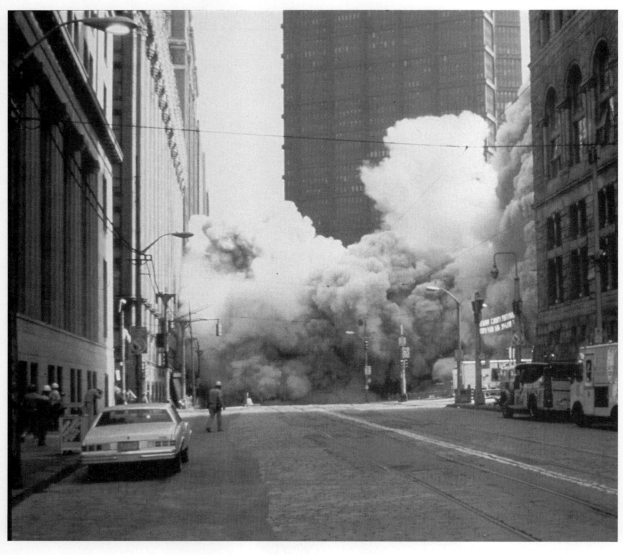

B. _____
   _____
   _____
   _____
   _____
   _____
   _____
   _____
   _____
   _____
   _____
   _____
   _____

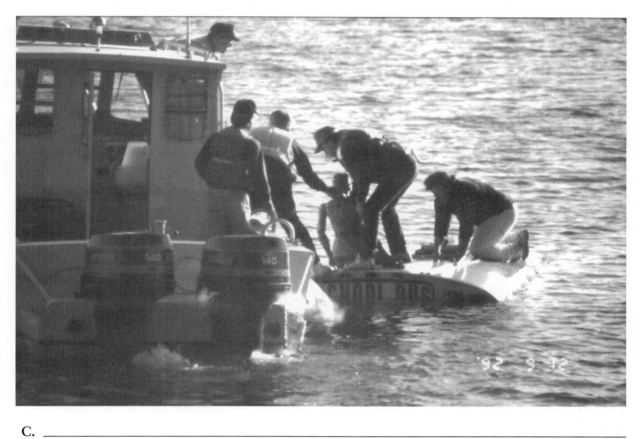

C. _____

_____

_____

_____

_____

_____

_____

_____

_____

_____

_____

_____

_____

_____

CHAPTER 3
Patient Assessment in the Field

Section II, pp. 200–232

Review of Chapter Objectives

After reading this chapter, you should be able to:

19. Describe orthostatic vital signs and evaluate their usefulness in assessing a patient in shock.

The test for orthostatic vital signs, also called the tilt test, evaluates vital signs (blood pressure and pulse rate) before and after moving the patient from the supine to the seated, then to the full standing position. If after 30 to 60 seconds either the blood pressure drops by more than 10 mmHg or the pulse rate rises by more than 10, consider the test positive and suspect hypovolemia. (Note that the change in pulse rate is the more sensitive indicator.) Do not use this test when other indicators of shock are present as it places stress on the cardiovascular system.

20. Describe the medical patient physical examination.

The medical patient physical exam evaluates the head, ears, eyes, nose, and throat (HEENT), chest, abdomen, pelvis, extremities, posterior surface, and vital signs discretely, looking for illness or disease signs. The exam may be modified to meet the specific patient complaints of chest pain, respiratory distress, altered mental status, and acute abdomen. The medical patient exam may also include the results of pulse oximetry as well as cardiac and glucose level monitoring.

21. Differentiate between the assessment for unresponsive, altered mental status, and alert medical patients.

Responsive and unresponsive medical patients are examined in much different fashions. The **responsive patient** can provide information regarding his or her chief complaint, history of the present illness, past medical history, and current health status. This information, along with a physical exam focused on the areas of expected signs, provides the information necessary to make a field diagnosis.

The **unresponsive patient** cannot provide this information, and the care giver must garner it from family and bystanders and through a more intensive and comprehensive physical examination.

The **patient with an altered mental status** is assessed like the unresponsive patient, though some information may be obtained from the patient. The information may not be reliable, hence the need for a more comprehensive physical exam.

22. Discuss the reasons for reconsidering the mechanism of injury.

After the initial and rapid trauma assessments or focused history and physical exam, you have gathered enough information about your patient to determine if the mechanism of injury (and your resulting index of suspicion for associated injuries) agree with your assessment findings. If they do, maintain your priority for care and transport. If they do not agree, reevaluate your index of suspicion and the physical findings and possibly adjust your patient's priority. If you do alter your patient's priority, always err on the side of precaution.

23. Recite examples and explain why patients should receive a rapid trauma assessment.   p. 202

Every patient with a significant mechanism of injury, an altered level of consciousness, or multiple body-system traumas should receive the rapid trauma assessment. These patients are likely to have serious internal injuries and/or hemorrhage. However, the signs and symptoms of serious injury and shock are often hidden by other, more gruesome or painful injuries or by the body's compensatory mechanisms. Without maintaining a high index of suspicion for serious injury and evaluating the patient via the rapid trauma assessment, you are likely to overlook the patient with serious and life-threatening injury.

24. Describe the trauma patient physical examination.   pp. 203–212

The physical assessment of the trauma patient begins during the initial assessment with the check of the ABCs and then branches to either the rapid trauma assessment or focused history and physical exam. The patient with a serious mechanism of injury, altered mental status, or multi-system trauma receives a rapid trauma assessment, a fast, systematic physical exam evaluating body regions where serious or life-threatening problems are likely to occur. This assessment is a rapid evaluation of the critical structures and regions of the head (HEENT), neck, chest, abdomen, pelvis, extremities, posterior body, and vital signs. The patient with isolated trauma has an assessment directed at the areas of expected injury or patient complaint.

25. Describe the elements of the rapid trauma assessment and discuss their evaluation.   pp. 202–211

Each region of the body is inspected, palpated, and, as appropriate, auscultated and percussed to identify the signs of injury (DCAP-BTLS and crepitation). For each region, the specific assessment considerations include the following:

Evaluate the **head** for any signs of serious bleeding and deformity from skull fracture. Also check for discharge from the ears and nose, for the stability of the facial bones, and for the patency of the airway.

Evaluate the **neck** for lacerations involving the major blood vessels and serious hemorrhage and possible air embolism. Examine the jugular veins for abnormal distention and palpate the position and any unusual motion of the trachea. Also examine for subcutaneous emphysema and then any evidence of spinal trauma.

Evaluate the **chest** for signs of respiratory distress, including use of accessory muscles and retractions, and any signs of open wounds. Also observe the motion of the chest. Chest excursion should be bilaterally equal and symmetrical. Palpate for signs of clavicular or costal fracture and subcutaneous emphysema. Erythema may be present, but the frank ecchymotic discoloration of a contusion takes time to develop. Auscultate the lungs at the mid-axillary line for bilaterally equal breath sounds.

Evaluate the **abdomen** for exaggerated abdominal wall motion, and inspect and palpate for signs of injury, noting rigidity, guarding, tenderness, and rebound tenderness.

Evaluate the **pelvis** for signs of injury and apply pressure directed posteriorly and medially to the iliac crests and pressure directed posteriorly to the symphysis pubis to check for pelvic instability.

Evaluate the **extremities** for signs of injury, distal circulation, and innervation.

Evaluate the **posterior body** for signs of injury, and be especially watchful for potential signs of spinal injury.

Evaluate **vital signs,** first to establish a baseline, and then to obtain other readings to compare to that baseline. Evaluate direct pupil response to light during the rapid trauma assessment, but evaluate the other pupillary responses during more specific and directed evaluation.

Gather a patient **history** while you perform the rapid trauma assessment. This should include the elements of the SAMPLE assessment (Signs/Symptoms, Allergies, Medications, Past medical history, Last oral intake, and Events preceding the incident).

26. Identify cases when the rapid assessment is suspended to provide patient care. pp. 202–203

The rapid trauma assessment is interrupted to provide patient care whenever you identify any life-threatening condition that can be quickly addressed. Just as you would suction the airway when you find it full of fluids during the initial assessment, you might provide pleural decompression during the rapid trauma assessment when you notice a developing tension pneumothorax. You might also administer oxygen to a patient who begins to display dyspnea and accessory muscle use during your chest examination. Other examples might include employing the PASG for the patient with the early signs of shock compensation and an unstable pelvic fracture found during the pelvic assessment or immediate provision of spinal immobilization upon noticing a neurologic deficit during the extremity exam.

27. Discuss the reason for performing a focused history and physical exam. pp. 213–215

The focused history and physical exam is the third step (following the scene size-up and initial assessment) of the patient assessment process. It is an assessment directed at the areas where the signs of serious injury or illness are expected. It also draws upon a quick history to identify information supporting a specific diagnosis and elements critical to the continued care of the patient. The focused history and physical exam takes you quickly toward determining the nature of the illness or the existence of serious and specific injuries. It is performed in different ways for trauma patients with significant injuries or mechanisms of injury, trauma patients with isolated injuries, responsive medical patients, and unresponsive medical patients.

28. Describe when and why a detailed physical examination is necessary. p. 222

The detailed assessment is a combination of a detailed history and a comprehensive physical exam either to identify or to learn more about the effects of an illness or injury on the body. It, in its entirety, is employed only when all other assessment and care procedures have been performed, most likely during transport to the hospital and then only for patients with serious trauma or disease. Since the seriously ill or injured patients require constant care, this assessment is rarely performed in the prehospital setting. However, portions of the detailed physical exam are frequently employed to examine specific body regions, looking for expected signs of illness or injury.

29. Discuss the components of the detailed physical examination. pp. 222–228

The detailed physical exam involves a comprehensive evaluation of each body region using the skills of inspection, palpation, auscultation, and percussion. It begins at the head and progresses downward to the extremities and includes the following:

Head. Inspect and palpate for any skull or facial asymmetry, deformity, instability, tenderness, unusual warmth, or crepitation. Look for the development of Battle's sign and periorbital ecchymosis.

Eyes. Carefully inspect the eye for shape, size, coloration, and foreign bodies as well as pupillary equality, light reactivity, consensual movement, and visual acuity.

Ears. Examine the external ear for signs of injury and the ear canal for hemorrhage or discharge.

Nose and sinuses. Palpate the external aspect of the nose and examine the nares for signs of injury, hemorrhage, discharge, and flaring. The nasal mucosa is rich in vasculature and may bleed heavily.

Mouth and pharynx. Examine the oral cavity for signs of injury and the potential for airway compromise. Notice any fluids or odors and examine tongue movement for signs of cranial nerve injury.

Neck. Briefly inspect the neck for signs of injury with special attention to open wounds and possible severe hemorrhage and air embolism. Palpate the trachea to identify any unusual movement and examine for jugular vein distention.

Chest and lungs. Observe the patient's breathing for symmetrical chest movement and respiratory pattern. Note any accessory muscle use, and auscultate and percuss for unusual findings. Look for signs of injury, and palpate for crepitation and tenderness.

Cardiovascular system. Look to the skin for pallor, and palpate a pulse for rate, rhythm, and strength. Auscultate for heart sounds, and locate the point of maximal impulse.

Abdomen. Inspect and palpate for signs of injury and rebound tenderness, rigidity, and guarding.

Pelvis. Observe the area, then place medial and posterior pressure on the iliac crests and posterior pressure on the symphysis pubis.

Genitalia. As needed, examine these organs for hemorrhage and, in the male, priapism.

Anus and rectum. If hemorrhage is present, inspect the anus and rectum and apply direct pressure to halt bleeding.

Peripheral vascular system. Inspect all four extremities, observing and palpating for signs of injury and skin color, moisture, temperature, and capillary refill to assure distal circulation.

Musculoskeletal system. Palpate the musculature of the extremities, feeling for differences in muscle tone and the flexibility and the active and passive range of motion in joints.

Nervous system. Evaluate the nervous system by examining the following:

- **Mental status and speech.** Assess the patient's level of consciousness and orientation and compare these findings to earlier ones. Note speech patterns and the patient's appropriateness of dress and actions.
- **Cranial nerves.** Test the discrete cranial nerves that have not already been tested.
- **Motor system.** Inspect the patient's general body structure, positioning, muscular development, and coordination.
- **Sensory system.** Test for ability to sense pain, touch, position, temperature, and vibration over the extremities, and as necessary, the dermatomes.
- **Reflexes.** Test deep tendon reflexes with a reflex hammer, noting heightened or diminished responses. Test superficial abdominal reflexes and plantar response.

Vital signs. Repeat the evaluation of the vital signs including blood pressure, pulse, respiration, temperature, and pupillary response.

30. Explain what additional care is provided while performing the detailed physical exam. pp. 222–228

Since the complete detailed physical exam is an elective assessment, any time a significant sign of injury or the patient's condition suggests a care step, perform that step. The same principle applies when a portion of the comprehensive physical exam is performed on a discrete body region after the focused history and physical exam.

31. Distinguish between the detailed physical exam that is performed on a trauma patient and that of the medical patient. pp. 222–228

The detailed physical exam for the trauma patient focuses evaluation on the areas where signs of injury are expected based upon the mechanism of injury analysis or the patient's complaints (for example, examination for signs of anterior chest injury when an auto steering wheel is deformed). The detailed physical exam for the medical patient is directed to the areas of patient complaint as well as those areas where the signs of an expected illness might be found (for example, an examination for pitting edema in the dependent areas with the congestive heart failure patient). The history component of the assessment also differs with trauma and medical patients. With the trauma patient, you may gather an abbreviated (SAMPLE) history, while with the medical patient, you may perform a more in-depth history evaluation as described in Chapter 1, "The History."

32. Differentiate between patients requiring a detailed physical exam and those who do not. p. 222

The patients who receive a complete detailed physical exam are patients with serious medical or trauma injuries. They receive the detailed physical exam during transport to the hospital after other important care measures have been employed. They represent a very small percentage of patients that you will treat because seriously ill or injured patients often require almost continuous care. *Portions* of the detailed exam will, however, be performed on many patients, and these portions will be directed at a body region where signs of injury or illness are expected. Patients receiving portions of the detailed exam include those with isolated injuries and those patients with stable medical problems. Seriously ill or injured patients may receive a detailed exam aimed at discovering significant signs of the pathology generally associated with cardiac, respiratory, vascular, abdominal, musculoskeletal, or nervous system problems.

33. Discuss the rationale for repeating the initial assessment as part of the ongoing assessment. pp. 229–232

The initial assessment, with its examination of mental status and evaluation of the airway, breathing, and circulation, contains crucial elements of continuing patient assessment. These components of the initial assessment can quickly tell you when the patient is suffering from a life-threatening or serious problem and can help you monitor the patient's need for care. For this reason, these components are an integral part of any ongoing assessment.

34. Describe the components of the ongoing assessment. pp. 229–232

The components of the ongoing assessment include reassessment of the pertinent elements of the initial assessment, focused history and physical exam or rapid trauma assessment, and vital signs and include:

Mental status. Quickly reevaluate the patient's mental status to determine AVPU status or level of orientation.
Airway patency/breathing rate and quality. Perform a quick check of airway patency and breathing rate, volume, and quality to assure respiration is adequate.
Pulse rate and quality. Quickly reevaluate the pulse rate, strength, and regularity to assure they remain within normal limits.
Skin condition. Quickly check the skin for moisture, temperature, and capillary refill to monitor distal perfusion.
Vital signs. Reassess blood pressure and temperature (along with pulse and respiration) and compare to baseline findings to determine whether the patient's condition is improving, deteriorating, or remaining the same.
Focused assessment. Quickly reevaluate the signs of injury/illness to identify any changes. This may include reevaluating pertinent negatives to rule out an evolving problem.
Effects of interventions. Repeat the ongoing assessment soon after any major intervention to determine the intervention's impact on the patient's condition.
Transport priorities. Based upon the findings of the ongoing assessment, either confirm or modify the patient's priority for care and transport.

35. Describe trending of assessment components. pp. 229–232

Trending of the elements of the ongoing assessment—comparing of sequential findings—will suggest whether your patient's condition is improving, deteriorating, or remaining the same. This information prompts you to modify your priorities for patient care and transport, and may ultimately cause you to modify your field diagnosis.

36. Discuss medical identification devices/systems. p. 208

Examine the patient's wrists, ankles, and neck for medical alert jewelry reflecting preexisting medical conditions such as diabetes, epilepsy, allergies, use of medications, and the like. Also check the wallet or purse for such information. This information may help you and the emergency department in prescribing care for the patient.

37. Given several preprogrammed and moulaged medical and trauma patients, provide the appropriate scene survey, initial assessment, focused assessment, detailed assessment, and ongoing assessments. pp. 173–232

During your classroom, clinical, and field training, you will assess real and simulated patients and develop management plans for them. Use the information presented in this text chapter, the information on patient assessment in the field presented by your instructors, and the guidance given by your clinical and field preceptors to develop good patient assessment skills. Continue to refine these skills once your training ends and you begin your career as a paramedic.

CONTENT SELF-EVALUATION

MULTIPLE CHOICE

_____ 1. The focused history and physical exam is conducted differently for the four different categories of patients. Which of the following is NOT one of those categories?
   A. responsive medical patient
   B. unresponsive medical patient
   C. pediatric patient with altered consciousness
   D. trauma patient with an isolated injury
   E. trauma patient with a significant mechanism of injury

_____ 2. Which of the following is NOT a mechanism of injury that calls for rapid transport to the trauma center?
   A. ejection from a vehicle
   B. vehicle rollover
   C. severe vehicle deformity in a high-speed crash
   D. fall from less than 20 feet
   E. bicycle collision with loss of consciousness

_____ 3. The decision to provide rapid transport of a patient to the trauma center is predicated upon either the mechanism of injury or the:
   A. blood pressure reading   D. ongoing assessments
   B. physical signs of trauma   E. none of the above
   C. pulse oximetry reading

_____ 4. If you arrive at your patient's side only moments after the accident, he or she may not have lost enough blood to demonstrate the signs of shock.
   A. True
   B. False

_____ 5. Which of the following body regions is examined during the rapid trauma assessment?
   A. head   D. thorax
   B. neck   E. all of the above
   C. pelvis

_____ 6. The "B" of DCAP-BTLS stands for:
   A. burns   D. bilateral injury
   B. bumps   E. bruises
   C. blemishes

_____ 7. Which of the following is NOT represented within the DCAP-BTLS mnemonic?
   A. contusions   D. crepitation
   B. abrasions   E. swelling
   C. burns

_____ 8. Scalp wounds tend to bleed heavily because:
   A. there is a lack of a protective vasospasm mechanism
   B. the hair helps continue the blood loss
   C. the close proximity of the skull permits blood to flow quickly outward
   D. direct pressure is difficult to apply
   E. both A and C

_____ 9. Subcutaneous emphysema is best described as:
   A. a grating sensation
   B. air trapped under the skin
   C. air leaking from the respiratory system
   D. retraction of the tissues between the ribs
   E. fluid accumulation just beneath the skin

_____ 10. Suprasternal and intercostal retractions are caused by:
   A. tension pneumothorax   D. flail chest
   B. subcutaneous emphysema   E. either B or D
   C. airway obstruction or restriction

_____ 11. To assure adequate air exchange for the patient with a flail chest, you should:
   A. perform a needle decompression
   B. assist ventilations with a BVM and oxygen
   C. apply oxygen only
   D. perform an endotracheal intubation
   E. cover the wound with an occlusive dressing

_____ 12. When assessing the pelvis for possible fracture, you should apply:
   A. anterior pressure on the iliac crests
   B. lateral pressure on the symphysis pubis
   C. firm pressure on the lower abdomen
   D. medial and posterior pressure on the iliac crests
   E. pressure to move the hips to the flexed position

_____ 13. Your finding that a patient is able to move a limb, but the limb is cool, pale, and without a pulse is consistent with:
   A. neurologic compromise
   B. vascular compromise
   C. both a vascular and neurologic compromise
   D. spinal injury
   E. peripheral nerve root injury

_____ 14. The "A" of the SAMPLE history stands for:
   A. alcohol consumption   D. allergies
   B. adverse reactions   E. none of the above
   C. attitude

_____ 15. With a patient who has a crushing injury to his index finger received when it was caught in a closing door, which form of patient assessment would be most reasonable?
   A. the rapid trauma assessment and a quick history
   B. the rapid trauma assessment and a detailed history
   C. a quick history and a physical exam focused on the injury
   D. a detailed patient history and a physical exam focused on the injury
   E. a detailed physical exam

_____ 16. While gathering the history of a chest pain patient, you will likely:
   A. attach a cardiac monitor   D. start an IV, if appropriate
   B. administer oxygen   E. all of the above
   C. take vital signs

_____ 17. The pain or discomfort that caused the patient to call you to his or her side is called the:
   A. presenting problem   D. chief complaint
   B. differential diagnosis   E. present illness
   C. field diagnosis

_____ 18. A patient statement that "deep breathing makes my chest hurt" represents which element of the OPQRST-ASPN mnemonic for investigation of the chief complaint?

A. O   D. S
B. P   E. PN
C. R

_____ 19. The jugular veins in a patient with normal cardiovascular function remain full or distended up to which of the following degrees of patient tilt?

A. 15 degrees   D. 60 degrees
B. 30 degrees   E. 90 degrees
C. 45 degrees

_____ 20. If you hear bilateral rales on inspiration when auscultating a patient's chest, you should suspect:

A. congestive heart failure   D. chronic obstructive pulmonary disease
B. bronchospasm   E. all of the above
C. asthma

_____ 21. In a patient who displays hyperresonance to percussion, you should suspect:

A. pleural effusion   D. emphysema
B. pulmonary edema   E. none of the above
C. pneumonia

_____ 22. Examine a patient for unusual pulsation of the descending aorta:

A. just right of the umbilicus
B. just left of the umbilicus
C. along a line from the umbilicus to the middle symphysis pubis
D. just beneath the zyphoid process
E. anywhere in the abdomen

_____ 23. Accumulation of fluid within the abdominal cavity is common in patients with:

A. hypovolemia   D. gastric ulcer disease
B. aortic aneurysm   E. cirrhosis of the liver
C. emphysema

_____ 24. A patient in whom unequal pupils are a normal condition displays:

A. Cullen's sign   D. accommodation
B. anisocoria   E. Bell's palsy
C. consensual response

_____ 25. Vital signs provide the assessing paramedic with:

A. a window into what is happening with the patient
B. an objective capsule of the patient's clinical status
C. possible indications of severe illness
D. possible indications of the need to intervene
E. all of the above

_____ 26. A pulse oximetry reading of 88 percent would indicate the need for:

A. aggressive airway and ventilatory care
B. only the administration of blow-by oxygen
C. only some repositioning of the patient's head
D. no care at this point
E. careful monitoring of the patient for further deterioration

_____ 27. The type of patient most likely to receive the most comprehensive assessment is:

A. the severe trauma patient   D. the unresponsive medical patient
B. the minor trauma patient   E. A and D
C. the responsive medical patient

_____ 28. Paramedics employ the complete detailed physical assessment at the scene:
   A. rarely
   B. occasionally
   C. frequently
   D. rarely in trauma patients, frequently in medical patients
   E. frequently in trauma patients, rarely in medical patients

_____ 29. Reflexes not likely to be tested during the detailed physical exam are the:
   A. clavicular   D. Achilles
   B. biceps   E. abdominal plantar
   C. triceps

_____ 30. Serial ongoing assessments will facilitate:
   A. reassessment of the patient
   B. revision of the field diagnosis
   C. changes in the management plan
   D. documentation of the effects of interventions
   E. all of the above

SPECIAL PROJECT

Cranial Nerve Testing—Personal Benchmarking

One complicated element of the physical assessment is the evaluation of the 12 cranial nerves. You must learn not only the skill itself but also how to perform it quickly in the field, often under adverse conditions. To help with this process, attempt to evaluate the cranial nerves on yourself. This can aid you in remembering both the steps of the process and the normal and expected responses. This exercise can also help you maintain this skill during your career as a paramedic.

To perform this examination, you will need a retractable ballpoint pen, a penlight, some cotton swabs, a large full-length mirror, some cologne or perfume, and, for some tests, a partner. Practice this exam a few times, then repeat it a day or so later until it becomes a natural procedure. Doing so will help you when called upon to check the cranial nerves in class or on a patient.

I Olfactory (smell): Review page 140.

Close your eyes and one nostril and then sense for various odors. Use a perfume, cologne, or other nonirritating agent. You should be able to recognize various smells through each nostril. *(This check is not often performed in the field.)*

II Optic (visual acuity, peripheral vision): Review pages 60–61.

Evaluate each eye for visual acuity by testing gross image recognition at about 20 feet. Look for the smallest item you can discern. *Use your visual acuity (20/20, 20/40, or whatever) as a benchmark against which to gauge your patient's visual acuity (his eyesight is either better, the same, or worse).* Then extend your arms, move them backwards, behind your line of view, and wiggle your fingers. While looking straight ahead, bring the fingers forward until they just come into view. The angle made between your fingers and the tip of your nose is the angle of your peripheral vision, usually about 180°. *Perform this test on a patient by placing yourself face to face with him, extending an arm on each side of his head behind his ears, then bringing your hands slowly forward while wiggling your fingers. Measure the point at which he first notices your fingers.*

III Oculomotor (pupillary responsiveness): Review page 141.

This response should be tested on a partner because it is hard to watch the motions of your own eyes. Inspect the size, shape, and equality of the pupils. A slight inequality may be normal. With the room otherwise dark, shine a penlight obliquely toward the pupil. The light should cause both the affected and opposite pupil to constrict briskly (consensual response). Then check for near response. Have your partner follow your finger as you move it toward his nose. Watch for the eyes to converge and the pupils to constrict.

III Oculomotor, IV Trochlear, and VI Abducens (eye muscle control): Review pages 141 and 144.

Again, this response should be tested on a partner or someone else, as you cannot watch your eye motion in the mirror and follow your finger at the same time. Test extraocular movement (EOM) by having your partner follow the tip of your finger while you trace an "H" in front of each eye. As you move your finger, watch the eye and halt lateral motion when the eye stops moving with the finger. Then move the finger up and down while continuing to watch the pupil. Assure that the eyes move together. In the field, any restriction of motion should suggest muscle paralysis or possibly entrapment by an orbital fracture.

V Trigeminal (facial muscles and sensation): Review page 144.

Test the trigeminal nerve function by clenching your teeth and palpating the muscle tone. For sensory testing, check for bilateral touch sensation on the forehead, cheek, and chin using a sharp object (such as the tip of a ballpoint pen with the ball retracted) and dull object (such as a cotton ball). Lastly, touch the cornea of the eyes with a few strands of the fibers of a cotton ball and expect an immediate blink.

VII Facial (facial features and eyelids): Review page 145.

Closely observe your facial features for general shape and symmetry. Then raise your eyebrows, frown, show your upper and lower teeth, smile, and then puff out your cheeks. Close your eyes tightly and attempt to open them with finger pressure. Any unilateral strength, facial droop, or asymmetrical movement may be a result of nerve injury (possibly Bell's palsy).

VIII Acoustic (hearing and balance): Review page 145.

Occlude one ear with a finger and lightly tap the fingers of the opposite hand near the open auditory canal. Hearing should be clear and bilaterally equal. *For a patient, whisper something softly in the nonoccluded ear and ask him to repeat it.* Then check balance by closing your eyes for 5 or 10 seconds and noticing your position in the mirror after you open them. You should still be standing straight, not wavering, and you should not experience vertigo. *The patient should not move around more than when his eyes are open.*

IX Glossopharyngeal and X Vagus (speech and tongue control): Review page 145.

Listen carefully to your voice and articulation of words while looking in the mirror. Your voice should not be hoarse (vocal cord problem), nasal in tone (palate problem), and should be clear and distinct. Say "aaahhh" and watch through the open mouth. The uvula and palate should rise symmetrically while the posterior pharynx moves medially.

XI Accessory (shoulder and neck muscles): Review pages 145 and 147.

Examine the positioning of the shoulder (trapezius) and neck (sternocleidomastoid) muscles for symmetry at rest. Raise each shoulder against resistance from the opposite hand *(have a patient raise both simultaneously)*. Then turn your head against resistance (using your hands) to the left, then right. Any unilateral weakness suggests nerve injury.

XII Hypoglossal (tongue): Review page 147.

Stick out your tongue and watch for midline projection. It should remain straight and not deviate. Then move your tongue from side to side. Again, the motions should be symmetrical. *Any deviation is usually away from the affected side.*

CHAPTER 4
Clinical Decision Making

Review of Chapter Objectives

After reading this chapter, you should be able to:

1. Compare the factors influencing medical care in the out-of-hospital environment to other medical settings. p. 237

Most health care providers function in very controlled and supportive environments. The paramedic carries out the skills of other health care providers, but he often does so in hostile and adverse conditions. Paramedics perform assessments, form field diagnoses, and devise and employ patient management plans at the scenes of emergencies in spite of poor weather, limited ambient light, limited diagnostic equipment, and few support personnel. The paramedic also must perform these skills under extreme constraints of time and often without on-scene consultation and supervision.

2. Differentiate between critical life-threatening, potentially life-threatening, and non-life-threatening patient presentations. pp. 237–238

Critical life-threatening presentations include major multisystem trauma, devastating single system trauma, end-stage disease presentations, and acute presentations of chronic disease. These patients may present with airway, breathing, neurological, or circulatory (shock) problems and demand aggressive resuscitation.

Potential life-threatening presentations include serious multisystem trauma and multiple disease etiologies. Patient presentation generally includes moderate to serious distress. The care required is sometimes invasive but generally supportive.

Non-life-threatening presentations are isolated and uncomplicated minor injuries or illness. The patient is stable without serious signs or symptoms or the need for aggressive intervention.

3. Evaluate the benefits and shortfalls of protocols, standing orders, and patient care algorithms. pp. 238–240

Protocols are written guidelines identifying the specific management of various medical and trauma patient problems. They may also be developed for special situations such as physician-on-the-scene, radio failure, and termination of resuscitation. They provide a standard care approach for patients with "classical" presentations. They do not apply to all patients or to patients who present with multiple problems and should not be adhered to so rigidly as to limit performance in unusual circumstances.

Standing orders are protocols that a paramedic can perform before direct on-line communication with a medical direction physician. They speed emergency care but may not address the atypical patient.

Patient care algorithms are flow-charts with lines, arrows, and boxes that outline appropriate care measures based on patient presentation or response to care. They are generally useful guides and encourage uniform patient care, but again, they do not adequately address the atypical patient.

4. Define the components, stages, and sequences of the critical-thinking process for paramedics.

pp. 240–244

Components of critical thinking include the following:

Knowledge and Abilities

Knowledge and abilities comprise the first component of critical thinking. Your knowledge of prehospital emergency care is the basis for your decisions in the field. This knowledge comes from your classroom, clinical, and field experience. It is used to sort out your patient's presentation to determine the likely cause of the problem and to select the appropriate care skills. Your abilities are the technical skills you employ to assess or care for a patient.

Useful Thinking Styles

- **Reflective vs. Impulsive Situation Analysis.** Reflective analysis refers to taking time to deliberately and analytically contemplate possible patient care, as might occur with unknown medical illness. Impulsive analysis refers to the immediate response that the paramedic must provide in a life-threatening situation, as might be required with decompensating shock or cardiac arrest.
- **Divergent vs. Convergent Data Processing.** Divergent data processing considers all aspects of a situation before arriving at a solution and is most useful with complex situations. Convergent data processing focuses narrowly on the most important aspects of a situation and is best suited for uncomplicated situations that require little reflection.
- **Anticipatory vs. Reactive Decision Making.** With anticipatory decision making, you respond to what you think may happen to your patient. With reactive decision making, you provide a care modality once the patient presents with a symptom.

Thinking under Pressure

Thinking under pressure is a difficult but frequent challenge of prehospital emergency medicine. The "fight or flight" response may diminish your ability to think critically to such an extent that you are only able to respond at the pseudo-instinctive level, with preplanned and practiced responses (like the mental checklist) that are performed almost without thought. One example of a mental checklist includes the following steps:

Scan the situation by standing back and looking for subtle clues to the patient's complaint or problem.

Stop and think of both the possible benefits and side effects of each of your care interventions.

Decide and act by executing your chosen care plan with confidence and authority.

Maintain control of the scene, patient care, and your own emotions, even under the stress of a chaotic scene.

Reevaluate your patient's signs and symptoms and your associated care plan and make changes as the situation changes.

5. Apply the fundamental elements of critical thinking for paramedics.

pp. 244–246

Form a concept. Gather enough information from your first view of the patient and scene size-up to form a general impression of the patient's condition and the likely cause.

Interpret the data. Perform the patient assessment and analyze the results in light of your previous assessment and care experience. Form a field diagnosis.

Apply the principles. With the field diagnosis in mind, devise a management plan to care for the patient according to your protocols, standing orders, and patient care algorithms.

Evaluate. Through frequent ongoing assessments, reassess the patient's condition and the effects of your interventions.

Reflect. After the call, critique your call with the emergency department staff and your crew to determine what steps might be improved and add this call to your experience base.

6. Describe the effects of the "fight or flight" response and its positive and negative effects on a paramedic's decision making.

p. 243

The "fight or flight" response is the intense activation of the sympathetic branch of the autonomic nervous system. Secretion of the system's major hormone, epinephrine, causes an increase in heart rate and cardiac output. It raises respiratory rate and volume, directs blood to the skeletal muscles, dilates the pupils (for distant vision), and increases hearing perception. However, the increased epinephrine may diminish critical thinking ability and concentration, impairing your ability to perform well in an emergency unless you raise your assessment and care skills to a pseudo-instinctive level, at which point acting under the pressure of an emergency becomes second nature.

7. Summarize the "six *R*s" of putting it all together. p. 247

Read the scene. Observe the scene or general environment for clues to the mechanism of injury or nature of the illness.

Read the patient. Observe, palpate, auscultate, smell, and listen to the patient for signs and symptoms. Assure the ABCs and obtain a set of vital signs.

React. Address the priorities of care from the ABCs to other critical, then serious, then minor problems and care priorities.

Reevaluate. Conduct frequent ongoing assessments to identify any changes caused either by the disease or by your interventions.

Revise the management plan. Based on the ongoing assessments, revise your management plan to best serve your patient's changing condition.

Review performance. At the end of every response, critique the performance of your crew and identify ways to improve future responses.

8. Given several preprogrammed and moulaged trauma and medical patients, demonstrate clinical decision making. pp. 236–247

With your classroom, clinical, and field experience, you will assess and develop a management plan for the real and simulated patients you attend. Use the information presented in this text chapter, the information on clinical decision making presented by your instructors, and the guidance given by your clinical and field preceptors to develop good clinical decision-making skills. Continue to refine these skills once your training ends and you begin your career as a paramedic.

CASE STUDY REVIEW

Reread the case study on pages 235 and 236 in Paramedic Care: Patient Assessment *before reading the discussion below.*

This case study describes a typical trauma patient. The paramedic's initial assessment suggests serious impact, but the patient at first demonstrates no signs or symptoms of serious internal injury. As assessment, care, and transport proceed, however, the patient deteriorates, requiring the paramedic to employ critical clinical decision-making skills.

Sue responds to a routine minor trauma call. After performing an initial assessment and a rapid trauma assessment, Sue decides that the patient does not meet the criteria for rapid transport to a trauma center. Sues's rapid trauma assessment suggests that Marcie has experienced only minor facial trauma and signs and symptoms supportive of that determination. The only point of possible concern is Marcie's inability to remember what happened. However, her hemodynamic status and vital signs support the field diagnosis of minor facial injuries. Her patient acuity is determined to be non-life-threatening. Sue decides the closest community hospital is a good choice to assure quick care for Marcie's injuries and cancels the county medevac helicopter.

En route to the community hospital, Sue performs an ongoing assessment (every 15 minutes for a minor injury patient). She discovers that Marcie is showing some signs of a CNS deficit. This causes Sue to reevaluate her original patient acuity and field diagnosis. The degeneration of Marcie's level of responsiveness alarms Sue. Through divergent thinking, looking for other causes of Marcie's presentation, she changes the patient acuity to life-threatening and her field diagnosis to increasing intracranial pressure. She will no doubt now monitor Marcie every 5 minutes and focus her attention on the signs of increasing intracranial pressure, diminishing level of consciousness and orientation, as well as a slowing pulse rate and rising systolic blood pressure. If oxygen has not already been applied, Sue administers it, the urgency of transport increases, and the destination is changed to a trauma center.

Because Sue carefully monitored her patient and employed good critical decision-making skills, Marcie did not go to a community hospital. If she had, she likely would have been stabilized and then transported to a trauma or neuro-center, delaying her time to critical surgery. Such ongoing monitoring of a patient along with the anticipation of possible responses will help you provide the best care possible for your patients. As this call ends, Sue and her crew will critique their actions and search for ways to improve the care they give for patients with similar presentations.

CONTENT SELF-EVALUATION

MULTIPLE CHOICE

_____ 1. Which of the following terms best describes the first paramedics of the 1970s?
A. field technician
B. prehospital emergency care practitioner
C. orderly
D. field attendant
E. field aide

_____ 2. The term describing the severity of a patient's condition is:
A. multiparity
B. epiphysis
C. tonicity
D. acuity
E. declivity

_____ 3. The paramedic's final determination of the patient's most likely primary problem is know as the:
A. field diagnosis
B. differential field diagnosis
C. chief complaint
D. improvisation
E. standing order

_____ 4. Which of the following is NOT a level of patient acuity?
A. life-threatening condition
B. non-life-threatening condition
C. potential non-life-threatening condition
D. potential life-threatening condition
E. both A and B

_____ 5. Which patient acuity level presents the greatest challenge to the paramedic's critical-thinking skills?
A. life-threatening condition
B. non-life-threatening condition
C. potential non-life-threatening condition
D. potential life-threatening condition
E. B and C equally

_____ 6. Which of the following terms represents a flow chart of patient care procedures?
A. protocol
B. standing order
C. algorithm
D. special care enhancement
E. proviso

_____ 7. A policy of administering nitroglycerin to a cardiac chest pain patient is an example of a(n):
A. protocol
B. standing order
C. algorithm
D. special care enhancement
E. proviso

_____ 8. A policy by which nitroglycerin can be administered to a cardiac chest pain patient without a physician's order is an example of a(n):
  A. protocol
  B. standing order
  C. algorithm
  D. special enhancement
  E. proviso

_____ 9. The major disadvantage to the use of protocols and standing orders is that they:
  A. apply only to atypical patients
  B. often do not permit the paramedic to adapt to a patient's unique presentation
  C. only cover multiple disease etiologies
  D. address only patients with vague presentations
  E. none of the above

_____ 10. In the case where a particular protocol does not seem to fit the patient presentation, you should contact the medical direction physician for advice and direction regarding your patient's care.
  A. True
  B. False

_____ 11. The data-processing style that focuses on the most important aspect of a critical situation is:
  A. reflective
  B. impulsive
  C. divergent
  D. convergent
  E. anticipatory

_____ 12. The style of situation analysis that causes you to respond instinctively to a situation rather than to think about it is:
  A. reflective
  B. impulsive
  C. divergent
  D. convergent
  E. anticipatory

_____ 13. One way to remain in control in otherwise extremely stressful situations is to learn to perform technical skills at a pseudo-instinctive level.
  A. True
  B. False

_____ 14. Which of the following is NOT a step in the critical decision-making process?
  A. forming a concept
  B. interpreting the data
  C. applying the principles
  D. summarizing the result
  E. evaluating the interventions

_____ 15. Which of the following is NOT an element of the six "Rs" of critical decision making?
  A. reading the scene
  B. researching the management plan
  C. reacting
  D. reading the patient
  E. reevaluating

MATCHING

Write the letter of the step in the critical decision-making process in the space provided next to the emergency response action appropriate for that step.

A. Form a concept.
B. Interpret the data.
C. Apply the principles.
D. Evaluate.
E. Reflect.

_____ 16. Field diagnosis

_____ 17. Provide ongoing assessment

_____ 18. Perform the focused physical exam

_____ 19. Pulse oximetry

_____ 20. Follow standing orders

_____ 21. Differential diagnosis

_____ 22. Assess MS-ABCs

_____ 23. Employ protocols

_____ 24. Determine the initial vital signs

_____ 25. Determine if treatment is improving the patient's condition

CHAPTER 5

Communications

Review of Chapter Objectives

After reading this chapter, you should be able to:

1. Identify the role and importance of verbal, written, and electronic communications in the provision of EMS. pp. 254–258

EMS is a team endeavor that requires effective communications among the various participants in the response and patient care. This communication is between you and the emergency dispatcher, the patient, his family, bystanders, other emergency response personnel, such as police, fire, and rescue personnel, and health care professionals from physicians' offices, clinics, and emergency departments, and finally with the medical direction physician. These communications, be they oral, written, or electronic, establish the key links that assure the best patient outcome.

2. Describe the phases of communications necessary to complete a typical EMS response.

Detection and citizen access pp. 257–258

This marks the initial entry point into the emergency service system at which a party identifies that an emergency exists and then requests EMS assistance through a universal entry number such as 911 or some other mechanism.

Call taking p. 258

This is the stage of EMS response in which a call taker questions the caller about the reported emergency in order to identify its exact location, determine the nature of the call, and initiate an appropriate response.

Emergency response p. 258

This phase includes the activities occurring from the moment a dispatcher requests a response by an EMS unit until the call concludes with the unit back in service. It includes various radio, face-to-face, and written communications among the dispatcher, emergency response crews, the patient, family and bystanders, and health care professionals, including the medical direction physician.

Prearrival instructions p. 259

These are a series of predetermined, medically approved instructions given by the dispatcher to the caller to help the caller provide some patient support until EMS personnel arrive.

Call coordination and incident recording p. 259

These terms refer to the interactions between the dispatcher and the responding units that assure an efficient and appropriate response. Call coordinating, for example, might involve changing the mode of response and the number and type of responding units. Incident recording refers to the logging of times associated with various response activities and the tape recording of communications associated with the call.

Discussion with medical direction
pp. 259–260

This is the opportunity for the care provider to describe the patient he or she is caring for and to obtain approval from the medical direction physician to initiate invasive or advanced life support procedures. Communication with medical direction also permits the emergency department to prepare for the patient's arrival.

Transfer communications
p. 260

These are the communications that occur between the first responder and the paramedic or as the patient is delivered to the emergency department. They are intended to communicate the results of the assessment, the care given, and the patient's response to care prior to the arrival of the paramedic or arrival at the emergency department.

3. List factors that impede and enhance effective verbal and written communications.
pp. 254–256

The factors impacting effective verbal or written communications are either semantic (dealing with the meaning of words) or technical (hardware).

In the area of semantics, the use of standard codes and plain English in verbal communications enhances good and clear communications, while use of nonstandard codes and jargon may confuse it. The same holds true for written communication. Nonstandard abbreviations and subjective, sloppy, incomplete, or illegible documentation leads to confusion and miscommunication. Complete, objective, legible, and efficient documentation leads to an efficient transfer of information. A well-designed prehospital care report makes written communication easier.

In the technical area, a well-designed and maintained radio or phone communications system will go a long way in assuring good and dependable communications. Improperly maintained or operated radios will, on the other hand, likely provide only intermittent and poor quality communication.

4. Explain the value of data collection during an EMS response.
pp. 255–256

The written call report is a record that includes the patient's name and address, scene location, agency responding, crew on board, and the times associated with response, arrival, and transport to a care facility. It also contains the results of the assessment and care of the patient. This administrative information can be used to bill for services and improve EMS system efficiency, by quality assurance/improvement committees to improve system performance, and by educators and researchers to identify what the system is doing and the impacts of its interventions. Finally, the call report becomes a legal record of the incident and the EMS care provided or offered.

5. Recognize the legal status of verbal, written, and electronic communications related to an EMS response.
pp. 254–256

The legal guidelines that apply to verbal and written communication in emergency medical service also apply to electronic communications. The information in these communications is considered confidential and must only be released in approved circumstances. The reports must be objective and not demean, libel, or slander another person. Any such action is accountable in a court of law.

6. Identify current and new technology used to collect and exchange patient and/or scene information electronically.
pp. 260–264

Cellular phones today provide duplex communications directly from the patient's side to the emergency department. These lightweight and versatile devices enhance EMS-to-physician communications and permit excellent ECG transmission. The only disadvantages to cell phones are user fees and unreliability at peak times.

Another electronic aid to dispatch is the facsimile or fax machine. It permits dispatch to send hard copy to the responding unit's station, assuring that elements of the address and nature of the dispatch are communicated accurately.

Computers are also increasing the efficiency of the dispatch system by recording times and system action in real time and making data recovery and research much easier.

Other new technologies that may affect prehospital care include: the electronic touch pad, which allows rapid recording of patient information; the handheld computer, which uses a pen-based system to log patient information and times associated with the emergency response and care; electronic transmission of diagnostic information (including pulse oximetry, 12-lead ECG, blood sugar, and end-expiratory CO_2 monitoring) provided directly to the emergency department, which may change the degree and number of field interventions permitted. In the future, voice recognition software may make real-time narrative recording of patient evaluation and interventions at the emergency scene and during transport a reality.

7. Identify the various components of the EMS communications system and describe their function and use. pp. 252–254

The emergency medical dispatcher (EMD) is the person who takes the call for assistance, dispatches the appropriate units, monitors the call's progress, and assures that the pertinent response data is recorded. He or she may guide the caller through initial emergency care using prearrival instructions.

The patient, his family, and bystanders are responsible for detecting the emergency, accessing the emergency response system, and relaying information about the cause and nature of the emergency to EMS system personnel. Since they are not trained in emergency medical communication, the responsibility of assuring good communications falls on the members of the EMS system.

Personnel from other responding agencies such as the police, fire service, rescue, and other ambulance services are also individuals who provide information important to assuring proper EMS response, and their input must be taken into account to assure scene coordination and optimum utilization of resources.

Health care professionals (aides, nurses, physician assistants, nurse practitioners, and physicians) at clinics, physicians' offices, and emergency departments are important people in the EMS system. They can provide invaluable information about the patient and the care he or she has had or should receive.

Finally, the medical director and medical direction physicians are significant resources for the prehospital emergency care provider. They are the individuals who extend their licenses to paramedics, thereby permitting them to practice prehospital care. These physicians also represent a body of knowledge of emergency medicine that may be tapped while paramedics are at the scene, en route with a patient, or at the emergency department for guidance regarding patient care.

8. Identify and differentiate among the following communications systems:

Simplex p. 261

This refers to a radio or communication system that uses only one frequency and allows only one unit to transmit at a time. With this type of communication, one party must wait until the speaking party completes his message before beginning to speak.

Duplex pp. 261–262

This is a radio or communication system that uses two frequencies for each channel, thus permitting two units to transmit and listen at the same time. This is similar to telephone communication, where one party can interrupt the other.

Multiplex p. 262

This is a duplex system with an additional capability of transmitting data, like an ECG strip, simultaneously with voice.

Trunked systems p. 262

These are computer-controlled systems that pool all radio frequencies and assign transmissions to unused frequencies to assure the most efficient use of available communications channels.

Digital communications systems pp. 262–263

These systems translate analog sounds into digital code for transmissions that are less prone to interference and are more compact than analog (normal voice) communications. This type of a system can be enhanced with devices like the mobile data terminal, which displays information such as street addresses, and can prompt the responder to send information like "arrived."

Cellular telephones
p. 263

These are part of a multiplex radio-telephone system tied to a computer that uses radio towers to transmit signals in regions called cells. The technology is inexpensive but can accrue substantial monthly charges; the transmissions may be interrupted by certain geographic features; and heavy use at peak times may limit access to the system.

Facsimile machines
p. 263

These devices transmit and receive printed information through telephone or wireless communication systems. Such a machine might give a responding unit a print-out of the nature and street address of the call or, possibly, detailed medical information about it.

Computers
pp. 263–264

The use of these devices in EMS is expanding rapidly. They are already helping to analyze data for review of calls and dispatches. Portable input devices, such as the touch pad and handheld computer, are being developed to permit recording of emergency response events in the field. In the future, paramedics may use computers with voice recognition software to complete prehospital care reports without paper.

9. **Describe the functions and responsibilities of the Federal Communications Commission.**
p. 268

The Federal Communications Commission (FCC) controls and regulates all nongovernmental communications in the United States. It assigns broadcast frequencies and has set aside several frequencies within each radio bandwidth for emergency medical services. The commission also establishes technical standards for radio equipment, licenses and regulates people who repair radios, monitors frequencies for appropriate usage, and checks base stations and dispatch centers for appropriate licenses and records.

10. **Describe the role of emergency medical dispatch and the importance of prearrival instructions in a typical EMS response.**
pp. 258–259

The emergency medical dispatcher (EMD) is the first person in the EMS system who communicates with the scene and possibly the patient. He or she begins and coordinates the EMS response and communications and assures data regarding the call are recorded. He or she also provides prearrival instructions to callers—for example, how to perform mouth-to-mouth artificial ventilation on an apneic patient—so that emergency care can begin as early as possible, thus helping to maintain the victim until trained prehospital personnel can arrive.

11. **List appropriate caller information gathered by the emergency medical dispatcher.**   p. 258

The information that is gathered by the EMD to determine the response priority and that is then communicated to the appropriate responding EMS service includes:
- Caller's name
- Call-back number
- Location or address of the event
- Nature of the call
- Any additional information necessary to prioritize the call

12. **Describe the structure and importance of verbal patient information communication to the hospital and medical direction.**
pp. 267–268

The verbal patient report to hospital personnel and the medical direction physician is essential to assure the efficient transfer and continuity of care. It consists of the following:
- Information identifying the care provider and level of training
- Patient identification information (name, age, sex, etc.)

- Subjective patient data (chief complaint, additional symptoms, past history, etc.)
- Objective patient data (vital signs, pulse oximetry readings, etc.)
- Plan for care of patient

For the trauma patient, the information and order of presentation is the same, although the subjective and objective information are modified to include mechanism of injury and suspected injuries.

13. Diagram a basic communications system. pp. 253–255

Basic communication is the process of exchanging information between individuals. A model for a communications system should start with an idea, followed by the encoding of that idea into useful language, sending the encoded message via a medium (direct voice, radio, or written), having another person receive and decode the message, and ultimately, receiving feedback from the original message.

14. Given several narrative patient scenarios, organize a verbal radio report for electronic transmission to medical direction. pp. 252–268

During your classroom, clinical, and field training, you will communicate with various elements of the EMS system, including dispatchers, patients, family members, bystanders, other EMS and scene personnel, and health care professionals, including medical direction physicians. Use the information presented in this text chapter, the information on communication presented by your instructors, and the guidance given by your clinical and field preceptors to develop good communication skills. Continue to refine these skills once your training ends and you begin your career as a paramedic.

CASE STUDY REVIEW

Reread the case study on pages 251 and 252 in Paramedic Care: Patient Assessment *before reading the discussion below.*

This case study discusses an emergency call and the elements of communications and, specifically, the radio communications between the paramedic and medical control.

This case study identifies some of the common and critical elements of communication essential to the emergency response. First, someone needs to recognize an emergency exists (detection) and then they must contact the emergency response system (access). The dispatcher must then receive the call (call taking), determine its nature and seriousness, and dispatch appropriate resources to deal with the problem (emergency response). The dispatcher determines the priority of the call by asking the caller a series of medically approved questions. The dispatcher, in addition, provides the caller with basic, approved first-aid steps to perform (prearrival instructions) until EMS reaches the scene to supply more comprehensive care. The dispatcher also coordinates the responses of any fire, police, rescue, or other service units needed to the scene (call coordination). The dispatch center records the pertinent information and times associated with the call for further review by the system administrator, the medical director, the quality improvement committee, researchers, or possibly by attorneys (incident recording).

Once at the scene and actively involved in patient care, the care providers contact medical direction to communicate the patient's condition and the care they have begun. This communication paints a clear picture of the patient they are treating. It may stimulate questions from the physician regarding the findings and patient care and may elicit orders for invasive actions, such as starting an IV line or administering medications. When the paramedic communicates with medical direction regarding orders for invasive actions, he uses the echo procedure, repeating back the physician's orders word for word to assure that both parties understand what is to be done.

The communications between the paramedics and medical direction also enable the emergency department staff to prepare for the arrival of the patient (transfer communications). In this case, the patient's condition is critical and time is of the essence. When the patient arrives, the hospital is ready for immediate surgery. While in this case prehospital and hospital care do not result in patient survival, support of the patient's vital signs provides organs that are used to prolong other lives.

Another factor to consider in this case study is the hardware necessary to the EMS response. The cellular phone makes communications from a bystander at the accident site possible, and the system is alerted quickly to the patient's plight. A system status management and priority dispatch system assures ambulances are close to the areas where response is needed and allows for coordinated responses. It also assures that red lights and sirens are only used for true emergencies. The enhanced 911 system uses a computer to determine the quickest route to the scene and provide the responding ambulance electronically with a printout of all the pertinent information needed to respond without taking the dispatcher away from the caller. The paramedics probably send an ECG to Dr. Doyle while they speak (multiplex), and Dr. Doyle can interrupt them as they deliver their report to ask questions (duplex). This hardware and a coordinated system of communication assures the best response and care for the patients of this EMS system.

CONTENT SELF-EVALUATION

MULTIPLE CHOICE

_____ 1. Essential participants in communications within the EMS system include:
A. the emergency medical dispatcher
B. the patient, his family, or bystanders
C. other responders, including police, fire, and other ambulance personnel
D. health care providers, including nurses, physicians, and medical direction physicians
E. all of the above

_____ 2. In general, the use of codes decreases the radio time and increases the recipient's understanding of the message, which has led many EMS systems to adopt extensive use of codes for their communications.
A. True
B. False

_____ 3. A radio band is a:
A. series of radios that communicate one with another
B. pair of radio frequencies used for multiplexing
C. range of radio frequencies
D. pair of radio frequencies used for duplexing
E. none of the above

_____ 4. Use of proper terminology in both written and verbal communications will:
A. decrease the length of communications
B. increase the accuracy of communications
C. increase the clarity of communications
D. reduce the ambiguity in communications
E. all of the above

_____ 5. Features of the enhanced 911 center include all of the following EXCEPT:
A. display of the caller's location
B. display of the caller's phone number
C. immediate call-back ability
D. a system of physician/ambulance interface
E. both B and C

_____ 6. The answering center for emergency calls that then transfers them to the appropriate agency for dispatch is the:
A. enhanced 911 center
B. PSAP
C. GPS
D. Emergency Routing Center
E. none of the above

_____ 7. The system that uses standardized caller questioning to determine the level and type of response is:
   A. priority dispatching
   B. system status management
   C. enhanced emergency medical dispatch
   D. prearrival instructions packaging
   E. dispatch triage

_____ 8. The role of the modern-day emergency medical dispatcher includes:
   A. priority dispatching
   B. prearrival instructions
   C. call coordinating
   D. incident recording
   E. all of the above

_____ 9. The report that occurs as you transfer patient responsibilities to the emergency department staff must include:
   A. chief complaint
   B. assessment findings
   C. care rendered
   D. results of care
   E. all of the above

_____ 10. A radio system that transmits and receives on the same frequency is called:
   A. simplex
   B. duplex
   C. triplex
   D. multiplex
   E. none of the above

_____ 11. Which radio transmission design permits the receiver to interrupt the caller while the caller is talking?
   A. simplex
   B. duplex
   C. multiplex
   D. trunking
   E. none of the above

_____ 12. The radio system that uses a computer to determine and assign available frequencies is called:
   A. simplex
   B. duplex
   C. multiplex
   D. trunking
   E. none of the above

_____ 13. Advantages of cellular communications in EMS include all of the following EXCEPT:
   A. duplex capability
   B. allowing direct physician/patient communication
   C. ability to handle an unlimited number of calls
   D. reduced on-line times
   E. transmission of better ECG signals

_____ 14. One of the paramedic's most important skills is gathering essential patient information, organizing it, and communicating it to the medical direction physician.
   A. True
   B. False

_____ 15. A standard format for transmitting patient information assures all of the following EXCEPT:
   A. communication efficiency
   B. physician assimilation of patient condition information
   C. completeness of medical information
   D. easier use of multiplex signals
   E. both A and C

_____ 16. All of the following are appropriate for good EMS communications EXCEPT:
   A. speaking close to the microphone
   B. speaking across or directly into the microphone
   C. talking in a normal tone of voice
   D. speaking without emotion
   E. taking time to explain everything in detail

_____ 17. It is important to press the microphone button for one second before speaking.
   A. True
   B. False

_____ 18. If the portable radio you are using is unable to transmit well from your location, attempt to:
   A. move to higher ground
   B. touch the antenna to something metal
   C. move towards a window or away from structural steel
   D. both A and C
   E. none of the above

_____ 19. The major difference between the medical and trauma patient reports is that the trauma format provides a description of the mechanism of injury and identifies suspected injuries.
   A. True
   B. False

_____ 20. The Federal Communications Commission is responsible for all of the following below EXCEPT:
   A. assigning and licensing radio frequencies
   B. establishing technical standards for radio equipment
   C. assuring the proper use of medical terminology in radio communications
   D. monitoring radio frequencies for proper use
   E. spot checking radio base stations for proper licensing and records

SPECIAL PROJECT

Documentation: Radio Report/Prehospital Care Report

The authoring of both the radio message to the receiving hospital and the written run report are two of the most important tasks you will perform as a paramedic. Read the following paragraphs, compose a radio message, and complete the run report for this call.

The Call:

At 1515 hours, your ambulance, Unit 89, is paged out to an unconscious person at the local baseball field on a very hot (97°F) Saturday. You are accompanied by Steve Phillips, an EMT, your partner for the day, and are en route by 1516.

You arrive on scene at 1522 to find a young male collapsed at third base. He is unarousable, perspiring heavily, and his skin is cool to the touch. The pillow under the boy's head (placed by bystanders) is removed, the patient's airway is clear, his breathing is adequate, and his pulse is rapid and bounding. One of the bystanders says the patient was playing ball and just collapsed. Another young bystander identifies himself as the patient's brother and states that "nothing like this has happened before." He says his brother is named Jim Thompson, is 13, and lives about a mile away.

The rest of the assessment reveals no signs of trauma. The assessment findings include: blood pressure 136/98; pulse 92 and strong; normal sinus rhythm as revealed by the ECG; respirations 24 and normal in depth and pattern (at 1527). The boy responds to painful stimuli, but not to verbal commands or to his name. Pupils are noted to be equal and slow to react. Oxygen is applied at 12 liters by nonrebreather mask, and the patient is moved to the shade.

Receiving Hospital is contacted, and you call in the following report:

_____

_____

_____

_____
_____
_____
_____
_____
_____
_____
_____

Expected ETA at Receiving Hospital is 20 minutes.

Medical direction at Receiving Hospital, the closest facility, orders you to start an IV line with normal saline run just to keep open. You repeat the orders back to medical direction and then begin your care. Your first IV attempt on the right forearm is unsuccessful; the second attempt on the left forearm gets a flashback and infuses well. You retake vitals. The patient is now responding to verbal stimuli, the BP is 134/96, pulse 90, NSR via ECG, respirations 24. The patient is loaded on the stretcher at 1537 and moved to the ambulance.

You contact medical direction and provide the following update:

_____
_____
_____
_____
_____
_____
_____
_____
_____
_____
_____
_____

ETA 10 minutes.

En route, vital signs (at 1545) are BP 132/90, NSR via ECG, pulse 88, respirations at 24. The patient is now conscious and alert, though he cannot remember the incident. The trip is uneventful, and you arrive at the hospital at 1557. You transfer the responsibility for the patient to the emergency physician and restock and wipe out the ambulance. You report back into service at 1615, grab a cup of coffee, and sit down at the hospital to write the run report.

Complete the run report on the following page from the information contained in the narrative of this call.

Compare the radio communication and run report form that you prepare against the example in the Answer Key section of this Workbook. As you make the comparison, keep in mind that there are many "correct" ways to communicate this body of information. Assure that you have recorded the major points of your assessment and care and enough other material to describe the patient and his condition.

Date / /	Emergency Medical Services Run Report	Run # 911

Patient Information	Service Information	Times

Name:	Agency:	Rcvd :
Address:	Location:	Enrt :
City: St: Zip:	Call Origin:	Scne :
Age: Birth: / / Sex: [M][F]	Type: Emrg[ ] Non[ ] Trnsfr[ ]	LvSn :

Nature of Call:	ArHsp :
Chief Complaint:	InSv :

Description of Current Problem:

Medical Problems

Past		Present
[ ]	Cardiac	[ ]
[ ]	Stroke	[ ]
[ ]	Acute Abdomen	[ ]
[ ]	Diabetes	[ ]
[ ]	Psychiatric	[ ]
[ ]	Epilepsy	[ ]
[ ]	Drug/Alcohol	[ ]
[ ]	Poisoning	[ ]
[ ]	Allergy/Asthma	[ ]
[ ]	Syncope	[ ]
[ ]	Obstetrical	[ ]
[ ]	GYN	[ ]

Other:

Trauma Scr: Glasgow:

On Scene Care:	First Aid:
	By Whom?

02 @ L : Via	C-Collar :	S-Immob. :	Stretcher :

Allergies/Meds:	Past Med Hx:

Time	Pulse	Resp.	BP S/D	LOC	ECG
:	R: [r][i]	R: [s][l]	/	[a][v][p][u]	
Care/Comments:					
:	R: [r][i]	R: [s][l]	/	[a][v][p][u]	
Care/Comments:					
:	R: [r][i]	R: [s][l]	/	[a][v][p][u]	
Care/Comments:					
:	R: [r][i]	R: [s][l]	/	[a][v][p][u]	
Care/Comments:					

Destination:	Personnel:	Certification
Reason:[ ]pt [ ]Closest [ ]M.D. [ ]Other	1.	[P][E][O]
Contacted: [ ]Radio [ ]Tele [ ]Direct	2.	[P][E][O]
Ar Status: [ ]Better [ ]UnC [ ]Worse	3.	[P][E][O]

CHAPTER 6

Documentation

Review of Chapter Objectives

After reading this chapter, you should be able to:

1. Identify the general principles regarding the importance of EMS documentation and ways in which documents are used. pp. 272–274

The principal EMS document, the prehospital care report (PCR), is the sole permanent written documentation of the response, assessment, care, and transport offered during an emergency call. It is a medical document conveying details of medical care and patient history that remains a part of the patient record as well as a legal document that may be reviewed in a court of law. The PCR may also be reviewed by medical direction to determine the appropriateness of your actions during the call and used by your service to bill the patient for services. Lastly, the PCR may be used by researchers to determine the effectiveness of care measures in improving patient outcomes.

2. Identify and properly use medical terminology, medical abbreviations, and acronyms. pp. 275, 277–285

Medical terminology is the very precise and exact wording used to describe the human body and injuries or illnesses. Proper use of this terminology turns the PCR into a medical document. However, if terms are misspelled or misused, they may distract from the document and confuse the reader about the patient's condition and the care he either has had or should receive. Carry a pocket dictionary, and only use words when you are sure of both their spelling and usage. The same holds true of medical abbreviations. They must be applied properly and have the same meaning to both the writer and reader. EMS systems should use a standardized set of abbreviations and acronyms to assure good and efficient documentation.

3. Explain the role of documentation in agency reimbursement. p. 274

Good documentation is essential for ambulance agencies that bill for services they provide. The PCR provides the name and address of the patient as well as the nature and circumstances of injury and illness. It also includes the care and transport provided. Without this information, the service may not be able to obtain reimbursement for services rendered and, ultimately, to afford to provide the vehicle, equipment, and personnel necessary to provide prehospital emergency care.

4. Identify and eliminate extraneous or nonprofessional information. p. 290

The ambulance call should be documented in a brief and professional way. The PCR describing it may be scrutinized by hospital staff, the medical direction physician, quality improvement committees, supervisors, lawyers, and the news media. Any derogatory comments, jargon, slang, biased statements, irrelevant opinions, or libelous statements will distract from the seriousness of the document and from acceptance of the preparer's professionalism.

5. **Describe the differences between subjective and objective elements of documentation.**   pp. 290–292

Subjective information is information that you obtain from others or is your opinion that is not based on observable facts. It includes the patient's, family's, or bystander's description of the chief complaint and symptoms, medical history, and nature of the illness or mechanism of injury.

Objective information is information you obtain through direct observation, palpation, auscultation, percussion, or diagnostic evaluation of your patient. It includes the vital signs and the results of the physical exam, including such things as glucose level determination and ECG monitor and pulse oximeter readings.

6. **Evaluate a finished document for errors and omissions and proper use and spelling of abbreviations and acronyms.**   pp. 287, 289–290

The PCR must contain all information obtainable and necessary for describing the patient's condition recorded in a clearly legible way. The report must be written so that another health care provider can easily understand what is being said and can mentally picture the scene, the patient presentation, the care rendered, and the transport offered by the initial providers. In many cases, what to include in the PCR is a judgment decision made by the care provider, though the report must contain an accurate description of the patient's medical or trauma problem and an accurate and complete history. Correct spelling and use of medical terms is essential and reflects the knowledge of the care provider. Proper use of abbreviations and acronyms can help make the PCR more concise; their improper use, however, may produce ambiguity, confusion, and misunderstanding in readers. Reread the finished PCR and check it carefully before submitting it.

7. **Evaluate the confidential nature of an EMS report.**   p. 300

Confidentiality is a patient right and breaching it can result in severe consequences. Do not discuss or share patient or call information with anyone not involved in the care of the patient. The only exceptions—as necessary—are administration, which may need information for billing; police agencies carrying out a criminal investigation; requests for the information under subpoena from a court; and quality assurance committees that may need the information (with the patient's name blocked out) for system review and improvement or for research.

8. **Describe the potential consequences of illegible, incomplete, or inaccurate documentation.**   pp. 287, 299–300

A legible, complete, and accurate PCR is essential to call documentation. The information in it must be easy to read thanks to both good penmanship and conscientious attention to detail. The report must describe all the pertinent information gathered at the scene and en route to the hospital as well as all actions taken by you and others in the care of the patient. Failure to create a thorough, readable PCR reduces the information available to other care givers and may reduce their ability to provide effective care. The document you produce also reflects on your ability to provide assessment and care and your professionalism in general.

9. **Describe the special documentation considerations concerning patient refusal of care and/or transport.**   pp. 296–297

Be careful in the documentation of a patient who refuses care and/or transport. While a conscious and mentally competent patient has the right to refuse care, his doing so may pose legal problems for care providers. Document the nature and severity of the patient's injuries, any care you offered, any care he refused, and document carefully the assessment criteria you used to determine the patient was capable of making the decision to refuse care or transport. Also document the patient's reasons for refusing care and your efforts to convince him to change his mind. If possible, have the refusal of care and your explanation to the patient of the consequences of care refusal signed by the patient and witnessed by family or bystanders or police. Advise the patient to seek other medical help, like his family physician, and to call EMS again if he changes his mind or his condition worsens.

10. **Demonstrate how properly to record direct patient or bystander comments.** p. 286

Direct statements by patients and bystanders must be recorded exactly as they were made and the key phrases placed in quotation marks. Treating the information this way is highly important because it identifies that the information is directly from the source, not an interpretation. Identify clearly the source of any quotation you include in a PCR.

11. **Describe the special considerations concerning mass casualty incident documentation.** pp. 298–299

Often a mass casualty situation calls for an atypical EMS response and unusual documentation procedures. Care providers rarely stay with a patient from the beginning to the end of prehospital care, and the time spent at a patient's side is very much at a premium. Hence documentation must be efficient and incremental. Document your assessment findings and any interventions you perform at the patient's side quickly and clearly. Many agencies or systems have their own forms such as triage tags that simplify the documentation procedure.

12. **Demonstrate proper document revision and correction.** pp. 289–290

Everyone makes mistakes during a health care career and during the process of care documentation. When this happens, it is essential to make corrections in such a way that there is no appearance of impropriety. If an error is made, draw a single line through the error and enter the correction and your initials. If the error is noted after the report is turned in, write a narrative addendum explaining both the nature of the error and the needed correction and assure that the addendum is included with all copies of the PCR. Correct errors as soon as possible after they are discovered.

13. **Given a prehospital care report form and a narrative patient care scenario, record all pertinent administrative information using a consistent format, identify and record the pertinent reportable clinical data for each patient, correct errors and omissions using proper procedures, and note and record "pertinent negative" clinical findings.** pp. 272–300

During your classroom, clinical, and field training, you will complete various reports, including prehospital care reports, on the real and simulated patients you attend. Use the information presented in this text chapter, the information on documentation presented by your instructors, and the guidance given by your clinical and field preceptors to develop good documentation skills. Continue to refine these skills once your training ends and you begin your career as a paramedic.

CASE STUDY REVIEW

Reread the case study on pages 271 and 272 in Paramedic Care: Patient Assessment *before reading the discussion below.*

This case study identifies some of the important considerations regarding the prehospital care report and its potential to support (or incriminate) a care provider who is called into a court of law. The scenario emphasizes the importance of good documentation as described in Chapter 6.

We seldom realize the importance others may place on our prehospital documentation. In this case study, Tom Brewster is surprised when, three years after a call, he is summoned to give a legal deposition about it. While this example speaks to legal reasons for review of documentation, Tom might just as well have been asked about the quickness of the ambulance response, the time he and his crew spent on scene, or specific aspects of the care he provided. While attorneys may represent the most feared interrogators to most paramedics, the EMS system medical director, quality improvement personnel, or administrative personnel might also ask for details of some incident months or years in the past. For these reasons, your accurate and thorough documentation of the emergency scene and the assessment and care you provide is of great importance to you and your service.

Tom was asked about his recall of the events of the call and the comments made by the patient. His prehospital care report provided enough information to prompt Tom to remember the incident, the patient, and the care he gave. He was fortunate that his documentation provided this information and that he could piece together the events of that response. It is likely that the patient's attorney would challenge Tom's recall after three years. Documentation of the patient's statement that he "fell asleep" would be a factor critical in determining the reason for the crash (ruling out medical causes). Tom was apparently thorough in gathering the patient history and recording it on the PCR because he was able to recall that there was no history of either diabetes or heart disease. Tom further benefited from performing a routine but complete patient assessment, including glucose testing and ECG monitoring.

This case study emphasizes the importance of preparing a prehospital care report that describes exactly what happened and exactly what you did. Had Tom used sloppy penmanship or subjective statements or failed to provide complete information, the patient's attorney would have been able to challenge Tom's objectivity and accuracy. As things stood, the report supported Tom's recall and evaluation of the patient's condition.

CONTENT SELF-EVALUATION

MULTIPLE CHOICE

_____ 1. The prehospital care report is likely to be reviewed by which of the following?
  A. researchers
  B. EMS administrators
  C. lawyers
  D. medical professionals
  E. all of the above

_____ 2. Which of the following is NOT an appropriate purpose for reviewing a prehospital care report?
  A. to identify a chronological account of the patient's mental status
  B. to learn about what calls other paramedics had
  C. to help detect patient improvement or deterioration
  D. to identify what bystanders and family may have said at the scene
  E. to determine baseline assessment findings

_____ 3. The prehospital care report may yield information that the quality improvement committee may use to identify problems with individual paramedics or with the EMS system.
  A. True
  B. False

_____ 4. The prehospital care report should contain all of the following EXCEPT:
  A. a description of your patient's condition when you arrived
  B. your opinions about the patient's attitude or social/economic situation
  C. a description of your patient's condition after interventions
  D. the medical status of your patient upon arrival at the emergency department
  E. response time to the call

_____ 5. If you have doubts about the spelling of a term when completing a PCR, use a phonetically close spelling; doing this may still convey the right meaning and will not reflect poorly on your professionalism.
  A. True
  B. False

_____ 6. Which of the following is NOT a time commonly recorded on the prehospital care report?
  A. call received
  B. dispatch time
  C. arrival at the patient's side
  D. arrival at the scene
  E. departure from the scene

_____ 7. Since your watch, the dispatch clock, and other timing devices are not often synchronized, it is important to record all times on the PCR care report from one clock or watch when possible or to indicate when different clocks are used.
   A. True
   B. False

_____ 8. Which of the following is NOT an example of a pertinent negative?
   A. no shortness of breath in a myocardial infarction patient
   B. no history of epilepsy in seizing patient
   C. clear breath sounds in a congestive heart failure patient
   D. a blood pressure of 90/60
   E. no jugular vein distention in a congestive heart failure patient

_____ 9. The recommended way of indicating the exact words spoken by a patient or bystander is to:
   A. underline the passage
   B. draw one line through the center of the word or passage
   C. begin and end the passage with quotation marks
   D. place the passage in parentheses
   E. none of the above

_____ 10. All of the following describe good documentation EXCEPT:
   A. complete   D. objective
   B. altered   E. legible
   C. accurate

_____ 11. The PCR is created by the paramedic as a personal record of what happened at the scene and during transport and thus its legibility to others is not important.
   A. True
   B. False

_____ 12. The benefit of check boxes on a prehospital care report is that they:
   A. assure common information is recorded for every call
   B. eliminate the need for a patient narrative
   C. address every chief complaint
   D. speed the completion of the narrative
   E. all of the above

_____ 13. When should the prehospital care report be completed?
   A. at the end of the day
   B. at the end of your duty shift
   C. once back at quarters
   D. shortly after leaving the hospital
   E. upon or shortly after transferring patient care at the hospital

_____ 14. Whenever possible, have all members of your crew read or reread the prehospital care report before you submit it.
   A. True
   B. False

_____ 15. What is the best way to add additional information to the prehospital care report after it has been submitted to the hospital?
   A. Search and make changes on all copies.
   B. Change only the original report.
   C. Create an addendum and add it to all reports.
   D. Never add additional material to the report once distributed.
   E. Send a memorandum to medical control.

_____ 16. Use of professional jargon in the PCR is an indicator of the writer's professionalism.
   A. True
   B. False

_____ 17. Which of the following is the best example of a subjective and possibly libelous statement?
   A. "The patient smelled of beer."
   B. "The patient walked with a staggering gait."
   C. "The patient used abusive language and spoke with slurred speech."
   D. "The patient was drunk and obnoxious."
   E. None of the above is a potentially libelous statement.

_____ 18. Which of the following is a part of the subjective patient information?
   A. chief complaint
   B. past medical history
   C. history of the current medical problem
   D. patient description of what happened
   E. all of the above

_____ 19. The portion of your narrative report that contains your general impression of the patient is the:
   A. subjective narrative
   B. objective narrative
   C. assessment/management plan
   D. SOAP plan
   E. none of the above

_____ 20. You should document a pediatric assessment in head-to-toe order, even though you may have performed it from toe-to-head.
   A. True
   B. False

_____ 21. Which of the following is true about the body systems method of assessment?
   A. It focuses on body systems rather than body areas.
   B. It usually addresses only the system(s) affected.
   C. It is best suited to screening and preadmission exams.
   D. It can be a comprehensive approach to documentation.
   E. all of the above

_____ 22. The term that describes what you believe to be the patient's most likely problem is the:
   A. definitive assessment
   B. clinical diagnosis
   C. assessment object
   D. field diagnosis
   E. none of the above

_____ 23. The management portion of your documentation should include which of the following?
   A. any interventions
   B. the results of ongoing assessments
   C. any changes in the patient's condition
   D. the patient's condition when care is transferred at the emergency department
   E. all of the above

_____ 24. Which of the following is NOT a part of the subjective information recorded on the PCR?
   A. vital signs
   B. past medical history
   C. review of systems
   D. chief complaint
   E. none of the above

_____ 25. Which of the following are elements of the objective information recorded on the PCR?
   A. your general impression of the patient
   B. the results of any diagnostic tests
   C. the results of the physical exam
   D. vital signs
   E. all of the above

_____ 26. Which of the following formats records the chief complaint, history, assessment, treatment, and transport information in that order?
   A. SOAP format
   B. CHART format
   C. Patient Management format
   D. Call Incident format
   E. none of the above

_____ 27. The most significant feature of the patient management format of documentation is that it:
   A. documents the chronological sequence of events and actions
   B. focuses exclusively on assessment findings
   C. uses a free-flowing narrative style
   D. is most frequently used for patients with minor injuries/problems
   E. none of the above

_____ 28. The call incident format for documenting an emergency response is best suited for which type of patient?
   A. the unresponsive medical patient
   B. the responsive medical patient
   C. the trauma patient with no significant mechanism of injury
   D. the trauma patient with a significant mechanism of injury
   E. both B and C

_____ 29. In obtaining a patient refusal against medical advice, it is important to:
   A. determine that the patient is alert, oriented, and competent to make the decision
   B. clearly explain to the patient the risks of not receiving care
   C. try to convince the patient to obtain care
   D. explain that if the condition worsens the patient should call for the ambulance or otherwise seek immediate care
   E. all of the above

_____ 30. If your ambulance call is canceled en route to the scene, you should:
   A. simply return to base
   B. write canceled on the front of the PCR
   C. note the canceling authority and time of cancellation on the PCR
   D. secure the name of the patient as well as any other information
   E. none of the above

MATCHING

Write the letter of the word or phrase in the space provided next to the appropriate abbreviation.

A. shortness of breath
B. acute myocardial infarction
C. positive end-expiratory pressure
D. normal sinus rhythm
E. nausea/vomiting
F. do not resuscitate
G. breath sounds/blood sugar
H. premature ventricular contraction
I. not applicable
J. nitroglycerin
K. intraosseous
L. weight
M. sexually transmitted disease

N. against medical advice
O. congestive heart failure
P. chief complaint
Q. left lower quadrant
R. electrocardiogram
S. to keep open
T. central nervous system
U. intracranial pressure
V. jugular vein distention
W. treatment
X. motor vehicle crash
Y. year old

_____ 31. CC	_____ 40. MVC	_____ 49. DNR
_____ 32. y/o	_____ 41. STD	_____ 50. PEEP
_____ 33. wt	_____ 42. NTG	_____ 51. Tx
_____ 34. CNS	_____ 43. LLQ	_____ 52. IO
_____ 35. SOB	_____ 44. BS	_____ 53. TKO
_____ 36. n/v	_____ 45. ECG	_____ 54. NSR
_____ 37. AMI	_____ 46. JVD	_____ 55. PVC
_____ 38. CHF	_____ 47. n/a	
_____ 39. ICP	_____ 48. AMA	

SPECIAL PROJECT

Documentation: Radio Report/Prehospital Care Report

The preparation of both the radio message to medical control and the written run report are two of the most important tasks you will perform as a paramedic. Read the following information, compose your initial and updated radio messages, and then complete the run report for this call.

The Call:

At 1832, medic rescue unit 21 is paged through dispatch and is en route to a one-car accident at the corner of Elm and Wildwood Lane. One patient is reported unconscious, and the fire department is also en route. You and your partner, Mike Grailing (a paramedic), arrive with the ambulance at 1845 and find that there are wires down, fuel spilling from the gas tank, and window glass around the scene. Bystanders state that the car swerved wildly, then hit the power pole. You notice there are no skid marks. You stand by, awaiting arrival of the fire department and the securing of the scene.

Once the scene is safe, your partner employs a jaw thrust with cervical precautions and applies cervical stabilization, while you apply the cervical collar (1850) and begin the assessment. You notice a break in the car's windshield and a small contusion on your patient's forehead. He is unconscious, has a strong pulse, and displays some respiratory wheezing and stridor. Assessment of the neck reveals a small welt but no other apparent injuries. The pupils are equal and reactive. Oxygen is administered at 12 liters per minute via nonrebreather mask, the patient awakens, and initial vitals (including a respiratory rate of 30 with audible wheezes, BP of 110/76, a strong pulse of 90, and oxygen saturation of 94 percent) are taken at 1852. The ECG displays normal sinus rhythm.

The patient awakes and asks, "What happened?" He states that he thinks he was stung by a bee. Two years ago he had a similar sting and reaction and has a kit at home that his physician prescribed for him. He is experiencing itching, and there are noticeable hives. He says he feels like "I have a lump in my throat."

Based upon protocol, you initiate the IV run TKO with lactated Ringer's solution in the right forearm using a 16-gauge over-the-catheter needle while the patient is being immobilized and moved to a long spine board.

Medical control is contacted and you call in the following:

_____

_____

_____

_____

_____

_____

_____

_____

_____

_____

_____

Orders for 0.3 mg epinephrine SQ (1:1,000) and 50 mg Benadryl IM are received and the medications are administered at 1855. Just prior to moving the patient to the ambulance, the patient is monitored and found to have the following vitals: BP 118/88, pulse 78 strong and regular, respirations 20 and regular with clear breath sounds, an ECG showing normal sinus rhythm, and a pulse oximetry reading of 99 percent.

The patient history, which is taken at the scene and during transport, reveals that the patient's name is William Sobeski, his age is 28, and he lives at 2145 East Brookline Drive in the city of Rochester. The patient denies any allergy, except to bee stings. He was stung by a bee two years ago and was rushed to the emergency department because he "couldn't catch his breath." He denies any headache, visual disturbances, and any numbness and tingling. He also denies taking any prescribed medications and has not eaten since noon. The patient requests Community Hospital because his sister works there. En route, vitals are BP 122/78, pulse of 68 strong and regular, respirations 22 and regular, and a pulse oximetry reading of 98 percent, all taken at 1902.

Contact medical control and provide the following update:

_____

_____

_____

_____

_____

_____

_____

_____

_____

_____

_____

ETA 10 minutes

The final vitals, taken just before arrival, are BP 122/80, pulse 86, oxygen saturation of 98 percent, and respirations 24 and regular with no wheezes. The ECG still displays normal sinus rhythm, and the patient is conscious and oriented. He states that the feeling of a lump in the throat is gone.

The trip is uneventful, and the patient is delivered to the emergency department at 1925. The patient care responsibilities are transferred to the staff, and the attending physician is given the final patient update. The vehicle is restocked, cleaned, and you are ready for service at 1955.

Using the information contained in this narrative, complete the run report on the next page.

Compare the radio communication and run report form that you prepared against the example in the Answer Key section of this Workbook. As you make this comparison, keep in mind that there are "many correct" ways to communicate this body of information. Ensure that the information you have recorded contains the major points of your assessment and care and enough other material to describe the patient and his condition to the receiving physician and anyone else who might review the form. Remember that this document may be the only record of your assessment and care for this patient. When you are done, it should be a complete account of your actions.

Date / /	Emergency Medical Services Run Report	Run # 911

Patient Information   **Service Information**   **Times**

Name:	Agency:	Rcvd :
Address:	Location:	Enrt :
City: St: Zip:	Call Origin:	Scne :
Age: Birth: / / Sex: [M][F]	Type: Emrg[ ] Non[ ] Trnsfr[ ]	LvSn :
Nature of Call:		ArHsp :
Chief Complaint:		InSv :

Description of Current Problem:

Medical Problems

Past		Present
[ ]	Cardiac	[ ]
[ ]	Stroke	[ ]
[ ]	Acute Abdomen	[ ]
[ ]	Diabetes	[ ]
[ ]	Psychiatric	[ ]
[ ]	Epilepsy	[ ]
[ ]	Drug/Alcohol	[ ]
[ ]	Poisoning	[ ]
[ ]	Allergy/Asthma	[ ]
[ ]	Syncope	[ ]
[ ]	Obstetrical	[ ]
[ ]	GYN	[ ]

Other:

Trauma Scr: Glasgow:

On Scene Care:	First Aid:
	By Whom?

02 @ L : Via	C-Collar :	S-Immob. :	Stretcher :

Allergies/Meds:	Past Med Hx:

Time	Pulse	Resp.	BP S/D	LOC	ECG
:	R: [r][i]	R: [s][l]	/	[a][v][p][u]	
Care/Comments:					
:	R: [r][i]	R: [s][l]	/	[a][v][p][u]	
Care/Comments:					
:	R: [r][i]	R: [s][l]	/	[a][v][p][u]	
Care/Comments:					
:	R: [r][i]	R: [s][l]	/	[a][v][p][u]	
Care/Comments:					

Destination:	Personnel:	Certification
Reason:[ ]pt [ ]Closest [ ]M.D. [ ]Other	1.	[P][E][O]
Contacted: [ ]Radio [ ]Tele [ ]Direct	2.	[P][E][O]
Ar Status: [ ]Better [ ]UnC [ ]Worse	3.	[P][E][O]

PATIENT ASSESSMENT
Content Review

CONTENT SELF-EVALUATION

Chapter 1: The History

_____ 1. The listing of possible causes of your patient's symptoms or chief complaint is the:
A. presenting problem
B. field diagnosis
C. differential field diagnosis
D. chief complaint
E. summary diagnosis

_____ 2. Making a proper first impression involves:
A. developing trust between care provider and patient
B. developing a positive patient/care provider relationship
C. establishing the professionalism of the care provider
D. calming and reassuring the patient
E. all of the above

_____ 3. Which of the following is NOT a recommended action during your introduction to the patient?
A. assuming a position at the patient's eye level
B. addressing your patient by a familiar name like "Pops" or "Dear"
C. dressing in a fresh, clean uniform
D. introducing yourself by name, title, and agency
E. using your patient's name frequently

_____ 4. Which of the following is an example of an open-ended question?
A. Does your pain increase with breathing?
B. Have you experienced this problem before?
C. Do you take any medications for your condition?
D. Does the pain radiate to your shoulder?
E. Where do you hurt?

_____ 5. Which of the following questions is an example of a closed-ended question?
A. Has this happened to you before?
B. How would you describe your pain?
C. What you were doing when this problem began?
D. What medications are you on?
E. all of the above

_____ 6. The interviewing technique in which you restate the patient's words is:
A. reflection
B. clarification
C. active listening
D. confrontation
E. interpretation

_____ 7. The interviewing technique represented by the statement to the patient that "You say you feel fine, but you seem uneasy and uncomfortable" is:
A. distraction
B. reflection
C. facilitation
D. confrontation
E. clarification

_____ 8. The pain, discomfort, or dysfunction that causes the patient to summon emergency medical service is the:
    A. primary problem   D. mechanism of injury
    B. chief complaint   E. none of the above
    C. nature of the illness

_____ 9. The absence of dyspnea in a patient experiencing chest pain would be an example of which of the OPQRST-ASPN components of the history of the current illness?
    A. O   D. AS
    B. P   E. PN
    C. T

_____ 10. The CAGE questionaire is used in questioning a patient about:
    A. alcoholism   D. "caine" family allergies
    B. chest pain   E. current medication use
    C. dyspnea

_____ 11. Which of the following represents a 10 pack/year smoker?
    A. 1 pack per day for 5 years   D. 1 pack per day for 10 years
    B. 2 packs per day for 5 years   E. both B and D
    C. 4 packs per day for 5 years

_____ 12. Which of the following previous family conditions is not important in determining the family history?
    A. asthma   D. allergies
    B. cardiac problems   E. hypertension
    C. traumatic death

_____ 13. The term "para" refers to which of the following regarding the obstetrical status of a female patient?
    A. the number of pregnancies   D. the number of living children
    B. the number of viable births   E. none of the above
    C. the number of abortions

_____ 14. The first priority in caring for a belligerent and intoxicated patient is:
    A. having friends and family present
    B. creating a calming environment
    C. having enough personnel present to restrain the patient
    D. assuring a safe environment
    E. using appropriate clinical judgment

_____ 15. Most patients comment on and remember the technical skills and abilities of the paramedics that treat them.
    A. True
    B. False

Chapter 2: Physical Exam Techniques

_____ 16. Hyperresonance would be discovered during assessment using the technique of:
    A. palpation   D. percussion
    B. auscultation   E. none of the above
    C. inspection

_____ 17. To evaluate a patient's skin temperature, it is best to use the:
    A. tips of the fingers   D. back of the hands or fingers
    B. pads of the fingers   E. none of the above
    C. palm of the hands

_____ 18. To evaluate tissue masses, it is best to use the:
  A. tips of the fingers
  B. pads of the fingers
  C. palm of the hands
  D. back of the hands or fingers
  E. none of the above

_____ 19. To employ deep palpation, apply pressure and sense using the fingers of only one hand, which will increase your sensitivity to masses, guarding, and other pathologies.
  A. True
  B. False

_____ 20. The thudding sound produced by percussing a solid organ like the liver is described as:
  A. hyperresonance
  B. dull
  C. resonance
  D. flat
  E. none of the above

_____ 21. Tachycardia is likely to be caused by all of the following EXCEPT:
  A. fever
  B. pain
  C. fluid dehydration
  D. hypoxia
  E. sympathetic stimulation

_____ 22. The process of normal inspiration is:
  A. an active action involving accessory muscles
  B. an active action involving the diaphragm and intercostal muscles
  C. active in its early stages and passive in its later stages
  D. passive in its early stages and active in its later stages
  E. passive

_____ 23. The pressure of the blood within the blood vessels caused by contraction of the ventricles is the:
  A. Korotkoff pressure
  B. systolic pressure
  C. diastolic pressure
  D. asystolic pressure
  E. atrial pressure

_____ 24. The pulse pressure of a patient with a pulse rate of 72, a blood pressure of 120/90, and a respiratory rate of 16 is:
  A. 18
  B. 30
  C. 72
  D. 90
  E. 120

_____ 25. The average blood pressure in a healthy adult is:
  A. 90/60
  B. 100/70
  C. 120/80
  D. 140/90
  E. 180/100

_____ 26. The normal respiratory tidal volume for a healthy adult is about:
  A. 100 mL
  B. 200 mL
  C. 500 mL
  D. 800 mL
  E. 1,200 mL

_____ 27. The systolic blood pressure represents a measure of:
  A. peripheral vascular resistance
  B. the cardiac output
  C. the viscosity of the blood
  D. the strength of ventricular contraction
  E. relative blood volume

_____ 28. Hypotension is defined as:
  A. a systolic blood pressure below 100
  B. a diastolic blood pressure below 60
  C. a blood pressure below 100/60
  D. either a diastolic pressure below 70 or a systolic pressure below 90
  E. a lower than normal blood pressure

_____ 29. To facilitate conduction of high-pitched sounds through the stethoscope bell, apply the bell using:
  A. firm pressure
  B. moderate pressure
  C. light pressure
  D. alternating firm and light pressure
  E. no pressure at all

_____ 30. In a patient with a weak and irregular pulse, determine the pulse rate by assessing the number of beats in:
  A. 2 minutes and dividing by 2
  B. 1 minute
  C. 30 seconds and multiplying by 2
  D. 15 seconds and multiplying by 4
  E. 10 seconds and multiplying by 5

_____ 31. The width of a correctly sized sphygmomanometer cuff should be:
  A. one half to one third the circumference of the patient's arm
  B. one half to one third the radius of the patient's arm
  C. two thirds the length of the patient's upper arm
  D. one third the length of the patient's upper arm
  E. either A or C

_____ 32. When taking blood pressure, deflate the cuff at a rate of:
  A. 2–3 mmHg per heartbeat
  B. 4–6 mmHg per heartbeat
  C. 5–10 mmHg per heartbeat
  D. 8–12 mmHg per heartbeat
  E. 10–20 mmHg per heartbeat

_____ 33. As the blood pressure cuff is deflated, the first pulse beat heard through the stethoscope represents the:
  A. Kussmaul sound
  B. diastolic blood pressure
  C. systolic blood pressure
  D. the pulse pressure
  E. the doppler sound

_____ 34. The pulse oximeter reading indicates:
  A. carbon dioxide levels in the blood
  B. inspired air oxygen levels
  C. expired air oxygen levels
  D. blood levels of desaturated hemoglobin
  E. arterial blood oxygen saturation levels

_____ 35. Cyanosis is caused by an increase in:
  A. blood oxygen
  B. deoxyhemoglobin
  C. dissolved carbon dioxide
  D. carboxyhemoglobin
  E. natural coloration overshadowing the red of blood.

_____ 36. The discoloration that represents a blue hue is:
  A. cyanosis
  B. jaundice
  C. sckophosis
  D. erythema
  E. carotanemia

_____ 37. A heavy and greasy scaling of the skin under the hair is:
  A. dandruff
  B. nits
  C. seborrheic dermatitis
  D. psoriasis
  E. none of the above

_____ 38. The bluish discoloration just behind the ears, suggestive of a basilar skull fracture, is:
  A. "racoon eyes"
  B. "Battle's sign"
  C. periorbital ecchymosis
  D. Cullen's sign
  E. either A or C

_____ 39. The dark opening in the center of the eye that constricts and dilates to regulate the amount of light falling on the optic surface is the:
  A. retina
  B. pupil
  C. conjunctiva
  D. sclera
  E. lens

_____ 40. The term for blood in the anterior chamber of the eye is:
   A. hypopyon
   B. hyphema
   C. conjunctival hemorrhage
   D. anisocoria
   E. nystagmus

_____ 41. The term for the common runny nose is:
   A. epistaxis
   B. otorrhea
   C. rhinorrhea
   D. rhinitis
   E. none of the above

_____ 42. The layer of tissue that covers the exterior of the lung and helps assure that the lungs move with the thorax is the:
   A. visceral pleura
   B. parietal pleura
   C. peritoneum
   D. pulmonary pleura
   E. perineum

_____ 43. A location where you are NOT likely to notice retractions during forced inspiration is the:
   A. suprasternal notch
   B. intercostal spaces
   C. supraclavicular space
   D. costal border
   E. both A and C

_____ 44. A finding of decreased tactile fremitus suggests:
   A. pneumonia
   B. tumor
   C. pulmonary fibrosis
   D. emphysema
   E. none of the above

_____ 45. Which condition is most likely to cause an area of the lung that is hyperresonant to percussion?
   A. pneumothorax
   B. pneumonia
   C. hemothorax
   D. pericardial tamponade
   E. friction rubs

_____ 46. The high-pitched continuous, almost musical notes heard during chest auscultation of the asthma patient are:
   A. rhonchi
   B. stridor
   C. crackles
   D. wheezes
   E. none of the above

_____ 47. The "dub" of the heart sounds represents which event of the cardiac cycle?
   A. ejection of blood from the ventricles
   B. ventricular contraction
   C. ventricular filling
   D. closing of the aortic and pulmonic valves
   E. closing of the tricuspid and mitral valves

_____ 48. The sound of turbulent blood flow through an artery is a:
   A. trill
   B. murmur
   C. friction rub
   D. bruit
   E. gallop

_____ 49. Which of the following abdominal organs is located, at least partially, in the right upper quadrant?
   A. gallbladder
   B. transverse colon
   C. pancreas
   D. ascending colon
   E. all of the above

_____ 50. An ecchymotic discoloration over the flanks is:
   A. Grey-Turner's sign
   B. borborygmi
   C. Hering-Breuer sign
   D. Cullen's sign
   E. none of the above

_____ 51. Assessment of the musculoskeletal system involves:
A. examination of the passive range of motion
B. examination of the range of motion against gravity
C. examination of the range of motion against resistance
D. inspection and palpation
E. all of the above

_____ 52. The movement permitted between the metacarpals and phalanges is:
A. abduction/adduction
B. rotation
C. flexion/extension
D. supination/pronation
E. both A and C

_____ 53. To test for carpal tunnel syndrome, acutely flex the wrist for one minute and expect to have the patient complain of:
A. sharp pain
B. numbness and tingling
C. a burning sensation
D. dull pain
E. crampy pain referred to axilla

_____ 54. The most frequently dislocated joint in the human body is the:
A. shoulder
B. wrist
C. hip
D. elbow
E. ankle

_____ 55. The most common sprains of the ankle are:
A. medial
B. lateral
C. rotational
D. flexional
E. extensional

_____ 56. Which types of motion are permitted by the cervical spine?
A. rotation
B. lateral bending
C. flexion
D. extension
E. all of the above

_____ 57. The bony projection of the axis (C2) that the atlas (C1) pivots around is the:
A. trochar
B. ischial tuberosity
C. olecranon process
D. odontoid process
E. none of the above

_____ 58. An exaggerated curvature of the lumbar spine is:
A. lordosis
B. scoliosis
C. kyphosis
D. spina bifida
E. none of the above

_____ 59. A bounding pulse quality would be reported as:
A. 0
B. 1+
C. 2+
D. 3+
E. 4+

_____ 60. Which of the following is NOT a sign of proximal arterial occlusion?
A. cold limb
B. pulse deficit
C. irregular pulse
D. poor color in the finger tips
E. slow capillary refill

_____ 61. The cerebral cortex is the center for which of the following?
A. rational thought
B. behavior
C. speech
D. language
E. all of the above

_____ 62. Pitting edema that depresses one quarter to one half inch is reported as:
A. 0
B. 1+
C. 2+
D. 3+
E. 4+

_____ 63. The term dysarthria refers to:
A. defective speech caused by motor deficits
B. voice changes due to vocal cord problems
C. defective language due to neurologic problem
D. voice changes due to aging
E. joint pain and stiffness

_____ 64. A patient who responds to stimulation only for short periods is termed:
A. lethargic   D. comatose
B. obtunded   E. none of the above
C. stuporous

_____ 65. A question about what a patient had for lunch tests which of the following types of memory?
A. immediate   D. remote
B. verifiable   E. none of the above
C. recent

_____ 66. The cranial nerve that controls pupillary constriction is which of the following?
A. CN-I   D. CN-VII
B. CN-II   E. CN-X
C. CN-III

_____ 67. There are how many cranial nerves?
A. 4 pairs   D. 12 pairs
B. 6 pairs   E. 16 pairs
C. 10 pairs

_____ 68. The cranial nerve responsible for the sense of smell is which of the following?
A. CN-I   D. CN-VII
B. CN-II   E. CN-X
C. CN-III

_____ 69. The cranial nerve that controls most facial muscles is which of the following?
A. CN-I   D. CN-VII
B. CN-II   E. CN-X
C. CN-III

_____ 70. When a person loses his sense of balance, which cranial nerve has probably been injured?
A. equilibrial   D. vagus
B. glossopharyngeal   E. accessory
C. acoustic

_____ 71. When your patient loses balance while standing with eyes closed, that finding is referred to as a(n):
A. positive Romberg test   D. negative Romberg test
B. expressive aphasia   E. vertigo
C. sensory aphasia

_____ 72. To perform the "tandem walking" test, have a patient:
A. walk heel-to-toe in a straight line
B. stand with eyes closed for 20 to 30 seconds
C. walk across the room, turn, and walk back again
D. do a shallow knee bend on each leg in turn
E. walk first on his heels, then toes

_____ 73. To assess the sensory system, you must test for:
A. pain   D. vibration
B. light touch   E. all of the above
C. temperature

_____ 74. Which of the following is NOT recommended as part of the assessment and care for an ill or injured child?
   A. Separate the patient from the parents if possible.
   B. Give the patient a toy or object to play with.
   C. Elicit a parent's help in obtaining a history.
   D. Perform invasive procedures late in the assessment if possible.
   E. Provide feedback and reassurance.

_____ 75. In what age group do children usually learn to walk?
   A. infant   D. school age
   B. toddler   E. adolescent
   C. preschooler

_____ 76. Which group of children is most worried about mutilation and disfigurement?
   A. infant   D. school age
   B. toddler   E. adolescent
   C. preschooler

_____ 77. Bulging along the sutures of the young child's skull suggests which of the following?
   A. meningitis   D. all of the above
   B. head injury   E. none of the above
   C. increasing intracranial pressure

_____ 78. Because of the cartilaginous nature of the thorax, young children are diaphragmatic breathers.
   A. True
   B. False

_____ 79. The normal systolic blood pressure for the preschooler is:
   A. 60 to 90 mmHg   D. 95 to 110 mmHg
   B. 87 to 105 mmHg   E. 112 to 128 mmHg
   C. 95 to 105 mmHg

_____ 80. The normal pulse rate for the infant is:
   A. 60 to 90 per minute   D. 100 to 160 per minute
   B. 65 to 110 per minute   E. 100 to 180 per minute
   C. 80 to 110 per minute

_____ 81. The normal respiratory rate for a toddler is:
   A. 30 to 50 per minute   D. 22 to 34 per minute
   B. 30 to 60 per minute   E. 18 to 30 per minute
   C. 24 to 40 per minute

_____ 82. Which of the following is NOT true regarding the abdomen of the child?
   A. The liver is proportionally larger than that of the adult.
   B. The spleen is well hidden beneath the rib cage.
   C. The abdominal muscles afford less protection than those of the adult.
   D. The abdomen bulges at the end of inspiration.
   E. Inguinal hernias are common in young male children.

_____ 83. The patient's current health status is recorded under which element of the SOAP documentation format?
   A. S   D. P
   B. O   E. none of the above
   C. A

_____ 84. The results of auscultation are recorded under which element of the SOAP documentation format?
   A. S   D. P
   B. O   E. none of the above
   C. A

Chapter 3: Patient Assessment in the Field

_____ 85. As a paramedic, you will frequently perform a comprehensive physical exam in the acute setting.
A. True
B. False

_____ 86. The component of the patient assessment process in which immediate life threats should be identified and corrected is the:
A. scene survey
B. initial assessment
C. focused history and physical exam
D. detailed physical exam
E. ongoing assessment

_____ 87. Which of the following is NOT a component of the scene size-up?
A. taking body substance isolation precautions
B. locating all patients
C. analyzing the mechanism of injury/nature of the illness
D. determining the priority for transport
E. identifying scene hazards

_____ 88. The personal protective equipment you should wear when planning to intubate a patient includes:
A. latex or vinyl gloves and a gown
B. protective eyewear, a gown, and a face mask
C. protective eyewear and a gown
D. latex or vinyl gloves, protective eyewear, and a face mask
E. latex or vinyl gloves

_____ 89. All of the following circumstances noted during scene size-up should lead you to expect more than one patient EXCEPT:
A. carbon monoxide poisoning in an apartment building
B. child seat and a diaper bag in a car crash
C. injury incurred during a tackle in a football game
D. twin spider webs in the windshield of a crashed car
E. hazardous spill in a high school chemistry lab

_____ 90. Two important functions that must begin immediately in the mass casualty situation are:
A. rescue and triage
B. fire fighting and rescue
C. triage and incident command
D. incident command and extrication
E. incident command and scene isolation

_____ 91. The initial assessment includes all of the following steps EXCEPT:
A. forming a general patient impression
B. gathering a focused patient history
C. assessing breathing
D. assessing airway
E. assessing circulation

_____ 92. The general patient impression is based upon all of the following EXCEPT:
A. patient gender and age
B. mechanism of injury
C. chief complaint
D. oxygen saturation
E. your instincts

_____ 93. During the initial assessment, you should stabilize the cervical spine:
A. immediately, if suggested by the MOI
B. after the airway is established
C. just before you attempt artificial ventilation
D. after the circulation check
E. as the last step of the initial assessment

_____ 94. A patient who does not respond to a painful stimuli is classified as which of the following under the AVPU system?

A. A
B. V
C. P
D. U
E. cannot determine with the information at hand

_____ 95. A patient who awakens to a loud shout is classified as which of the following under the AVPU system?

A. A
B. V
C. P
D. U
E. cannot determine with the information at hand

_____ 96. If your patient is responsive and can speak clearly, you can assume that his airway is patent.

A. True
B. False

_____ 97. The presence of a carotid pulse suggests that the systolic blood pressure is at least:

A. 60 mmHg
B. 70 mmHg
C. 80 mmHg
D. 100 mmHg
E. 120 mmHg

_____ 98. The focused history and physical exam is conducted differently for the four major categories of patients. Which of the following is NOT one of those categories?

A. trauma patient with an isolated injury
B. trauma patient with altered LOC/significant MOI
C. pediatric patient with altered consciousness
D. responsive medical patient
E. unresponsive medical patient

_____ 99. Which of the following is NOT a mechanism of injury that calls for rapid transport to the trauma center?

A. fall from greater than 20 feet
B. moderate vehicle deformity
C. death of another vehicle occupant
D. penetration of trunk or head
E. motorcycle crash

_____ 100. If you arrive at your patient's side only moments after the accident, he or she may not have bled enough to demonstrate the signs of progressive head injury.

A. True
B. False

_____ 101. Assume your patient has a spinal injury if you find:

A. a significant mechanism of injury
B. an injury above the shoulders
C. complaints of numbness
D. pain along the spinal column
E. all of the above

_____ 102. The "C" of DCAP-BTLS stands for:

A. cuts
B. cutaneous injury
C. circulatory deficit
D. contusions
E. carotid bruits

_____ 103. Fracture and manipulation of the clavicle are likely to lead to:

A. subclavian artery injury
B. subclavian vein injury
C. hemothorax
D. pneumothorax
E. all of the above

_____ 104. During the rapid trauma assessment it is important to carefully evaluate the abdomen to determine the exact nature of injury and then take the necessary care steps.

A. True
B. False

_____ 105. The "P" of the SAMPLE history stands for:
  A. past medical history
  B. palpated deformities
  C. precipitating factors
  D. pulse deficits
  E. pupillary responses

_____ 106. The field diagnosis for a medical patient is most frequently determined from:
  A. the physical assessment
  B. the patient's story
  C. the SAMPLE history
  D. the vital signs
  E. none of the above

_____ 107. Which of the following is a part of the patient history?
  A. chief complaint
  B. history of the present illness
  C. past medical history
  D. current health status
  E. all of the above

_____ 108. A patient statement that "he has substernal and left arm pain" would fall under what element of the OPQRST-ASPN mnemonic for investigation of the chief complaint?
  A. O
  B. P
  C. R
  D. S
  E. PN

_____ 109. Which of the following is NOT likely to cause jugular vein distention?
  A. cardiac tamponade
  B. tension pneumothorax
  C. right heart failure
  D. hemothorax
  E. all of the above may cause distention

_____ 110. If you hear diffuse expiratory wheezing while auscultating a patient's chest, you should suspect:
  A. congestive heart failure
  B. pulmonary edema
  C. asthma
  D. pulmonary embolism
  E. all of the above

_____ 111. The ECG allows you to determine all of the following EXCEPT:
  A. cardiac rate
  B. cardiac rhythm
  C. cardiac output
  D. sequencing of the cardiac events
  E. all of the above can be determined by the ECG

_____ 112. Which of the following patients is likely to receive the most comprehensive assessment?
  A. the trauma patient with a significant mechanism of injury
  B. the trauma patient with an isolated injury
  C. the unresponsive medical patient
  D. the responsive medical patient
  E. any unconscious patient

_____ 113. You would normally expect to perform the detailed physical assessment on the serious trauma or medical patient:
  A. early in on-scene assessment and care
  B. en route to the hospital
  C. late in on-scene assessment and care
  D. on-scene for medical patients only
  E. never

Chapter 4: Clinical Decision Making

_____ 114. The paramedics of the 21st century will be highly trained and practiced field technicians working under rigid protocols.
  A. True
  B. False

_____ 115. Which of the following is NOT a level of patient acuity?
  A. critically life-threatening condition
  B. non-life-threatening condition
  C. potentially non-life-threatening condition
  D. potentially life-threatening condition
  E. none of the above

_____ 116. A standard of emergency care approved by the system medical director is a(n):
  A. protocol
  B. standing order
  C. algorithm
  D. special care enhancement
  E. none of the above

_____ 117. To employ critical decision-making skills as a paramedic, you must first have an:
  A. excellent working knowledge of pathophysiology
  B. excellent working knowledge of anatomy and physiology
  C. understanding of the role each body system plays in overall body function
  D. ability to analyze numerous signs and symptoms associated with the disease
  E. all of the above

_____ 118. The key to remaining calm and functioning well under the stress of an emergency is to:
  A. focus on the task and block out distractions
  B. let others know you are struggling and need help
  C. stay away from a systematic approach as emergencies are usually unanticipated
  D. employ one management style and stick with it
  E. all of the above

_____ 119. The thinking style in which all aspects of a situation are considered before arriving at a solution is:
  A. reflective
  B. impulsive
  C. divergent
  D. convergent
  E. anticipatory

_____ 120. The body system that may interfere with your ability to critically think at the emergency scene is the:
  A. cardiovascular system
  B. respiratory system
  C. somatic nervous system
  D. autonomic nervous system
  E. renal system

_____ 121. The portion of the mental checklist approach to emergency care in which you consider all options before employing an emergency care modality is:
  A. scan the situation
  B. stop and think
  C. decide and act
  D. maintain control
  E. reevaluate

Chapter 5: Communications

_____ 122. The basic communications model of exchange of information includes which of the following?
  A. sender encoding a message
  B. sender transmitting a message
  C. receiver decoding a message
  D. receiver providing feedback
  E. all of the above

_____ 123. The radio band that penetrates buildings and is less susceptible to interference is:
  A. VHF low-band
  B. VHF high-band
  C. UHF
  D. microwave bands
  E. none of the above

_____ 124. The prehospital care report should NOT be used by:
   A. administration for billing
   B. the emergency department staff to identify your patient findings
   C. quality assurance committees to improve system function
   D. other paramedics to identify your interesting calls
   E. insurance companies for billing

_____ 125. The phase of the emergency communications system that uses the telephone most heavily is:
   A. detection and citizen access
   B. the emergency response
   C. call coordination and incident recording
   D. discussion with medical direction
   E. transfer communications

_____ 126. The system that uses caller questioning and established guidelines to determine the types of units that respond to a particular emergency is:
   A. system status management   D. EMD
   B. priority dispatching   E. none of the above
   C. code identification

_____ 127. The radio transmission design that does not permit the receiver to interrupt the caller while he is talking is:
   A. simplex   D. trunking
   B. duplex   E. none of the above
   C. multiplex

_____ 128. Which of the following is NOT true regarding digital communication?
   A. It is clearer than analog.
   B. It is faster than analog.
   C. It may increase overcrowding of radio frequencies.
   D. It cannot be monitored by a standard scanner.
   E. It is becoming increasingly popular for EMS communications.

_____ 129. All of the following are appropriate for good emergency medical services communications EXCEPT:
   A. speaking close to the microphone
   B. speaking across or directly into the microphone
   C. talking in a loud voice
   D. speaking without emotion
   E. avoiding use of slang or profanity

_____ 130. The term for repeating an important order to assure it is understood correctly is:
   A. redundancy   D. reiteration
   B. multiplexing   E. either B or D
   C. the echo procedure

_____ 131. The Federal Communications Commission is responsible for all of the following EXCEPT:
   A. assigning and licensing radio frequencies
   B. establishing technical standards for radio equipment
   C. monitoring radio frequencies for proper use
   D. formulating acceptable medical information formats
   E. spot-checking radio base stations for proper licensing and records

_____ 132. The prehospital care report should contain all of the following EXCEPT:
    A. a description of your patient's condition when you arrived
    B. a description of your patient's condition after interventions
    C. the medical status of your patient upon arrival at the emergency department
    D. subjective opinions about the patient's dress or actions
    E. all of the above

_____ 133. Which of the following abbreviations represents patient history?
    A. PE   D. Hx
    B. HH   E. A and D
    C. H

_____ 134. Which of the following abbreviations represents alcohol use by the patient?
    A. AOB   D. OH +
    B. ASHD   E. none of the above
    C. ETOH

_____ 135. Which of the following abbreviations is an indication for administering something as needed?
    A. a.c.   D. prn
    B. stat   E. WNL
    C. npo

_____ 136. Which of the following is NOT an example of a pertinent negative?
    A. no respiratory distress in an MI patient
    B. nonreactive pupils in a head injury patient
    C. clear breath sounds in a congestive heart failure patient
    D. no history of epilepsy in seizing patient
    E. no pitting edema in a congestive heart failure patient

_____ 137. It is better to rephrase a patient's statement regarding history or a symptom, making it more medically correct, than to report it verbatim.
    A. True
    B. False

_____ 138. The best time and place to complete the prehospital report form is:
    A. at the scene, if possible
    B. in the ambulance, en route to the hospital
    C. at the hospital before you end patient care
    D. at the hospital after you end patient care
    E. at the station after the call

_____ 139. The best way to add additional information to the prehospital care report after it has been submitted to the hospital is to:
    A. search and make changes on all copies
    B. change only the original report
    C. create an addendum and add it to all reports
    D. never add any additional material to the report once submitted
    E. make notes only on your personal copy for future reference

_____ 140. The recommended way of making a correction to the prehospital care report is to:
    A. draw a line through the error and initial it
    B. erase the error completely
    C. draw up a new form
    D. blacken the error so it is unreadable
    E. any of the above are acceptable

_____ 141. Which of the following is subjective patient information?
   A. mechanism of injury   D. signs of injury
   B. past medical history   E. all of the above
   C. blood pressure

_____ 142. Which of the following is objective patient information?
   A. chief complaint   D. patient description of what happened
   B. past medical history   E. all of the above
   C. vital signs

_____ 143. The statement "possible angina" in the assessment management section of a PCR is best described as:
   A. the patient's presenting problem   D. a pertinent negative
   B. the differential field diagnosis   E. both A and C
   C. the field diagnosis

_____ 144. Under which element of the SOAP format would you place the patient's chief complaint?
   A. subjective   D. plan
   B. objective   E. none of the above
   C. assessment

_____ 145. Under which element of the SOAP format would you place your field diagnosis?
   A. subjective   D. plan
   B. objective   E. none of the above
   C. assessment

_____ 146. Under which element of the CHART format would you place standing orders?
   A. C   D. R
   B. H   E. T
   C. A

_____ 147. The system of documentation that records information based upon time and sequence of events is the:
   A. SOAP format   D. call incident approach
   B. CHART format   E. either B or D
   C. patient management format

_____ 148. When a patient refuses care against your advice, you must be sure to document that:
   A. the patient is alert, oriented, and competent to make the decision.
   B. you have clearly explained the risks of not receiving care
   C. you have tried to convince the patient to obtain care
   D. you have explained that if the condition worsens the patient should seek immediate care
   E. all of the above

_____ 149. If you arrive at the scene of a call and are told that your services are not needed, you should:
   A. simply return to service, with no need to complete a prehospital care report
   B. simply write "not needed" on the front of the PCR
   C. identify any canceling authority and the time on the PCR
   D. secure the name of the patient as well as any other information such as the SAMPLE history
   E. all of the above

_____ 150. Triage tags used for the mass casualty incident usually record:
   A. vital patient information
   B. patient priority for care and transport
   C. all minor injuries
   D. hospital destination
   E. both A and B

SPECIAL PROJECTS

Locating Auscultation Points

On the illustration below, identify where you would locate the stethoscope disk or bell to auscultate breath and heart (pulmonic, aortic, mitral, and tricuspid areas and PMI) sounds.

Fill in the Blanks

Explain the meanings of the following standard medical abbreviations.

1. CC   _____

2. HPI   _____

3. SOB   _____

4. ASHD   _____

5. HBV   _____

6. PND   _____

7. NTG   _____

8. PAL   _____

9. CBC   _____

10. PMI   _____

11. A/O   _____

12. p/y _____

13. WNL _____

14. BVM _____

15. ETT _____

16. NPO _____

17. Rx _____

18. KVO _____

19. SQ _____

20. BBB _____

Crossword Puzzle

Across

2. A rapid heartbeat
5. A wound
8. High-pitched respiratory sounds
9. Related to the heart
11. _____ complaint: the reason the patient called EMS
14. Fluid build-up in the abdomen
15. Written defamation of another person
16. Type of respirator used when treating a suspected tuberculosis patient
18. Involuntary response to a stimulus
19. Acute alteration in mental function
20. Loud, high-pitched inspiratory wheeze
21. Elements of the head assessment (abbr.)
22. Advanced life support (abbr.)

Down

1. Repeat a verbal order
2. _____ volume: normal respiratory volume
3. Basic EMS communication device
4. Against medical advice (abbr.)
6. Vomitus
7. Sound indicating turbulent blood flow
9. Light, popping nonmusical inspiratory sounds
10. Type of phone service used by many EMS systems
11. Grating sensation or sound
12. _____ diagnosis; prehospital evaluation of the patient's condition and its causes
13. Questionnaire used for suspected alcoholic patients
17. Severity of an injury or illness
18. Review of the systems (abbr.)

WORKBOOK ANSWER KEY

Note: Throughout Answer Key, textbook page references are shown in italic.

CHAPTER 1: The History

CONTENT SELF-EVALUATION

MULTIPLE CHOICE

1.	D	*p. 5*	8.	B	*p. 9*	15.	E	*p. 15*
2.	A	*p. 6*	9.	B	*p. 7*	16.	C	*p. 15*
3.	A	*p. 6*	10.	B	*p. 10*	17.	D	*p. 15*
4.	C	*p. 5*	11.	B	*p. 11*	18.	B	*p. 18*
5.	A	*p. 8*	12.	A	*p. 12*	19.	A	*p. 19*
6.	C	*p. 8*	13.	B	*p. 12*	20.	A	*p. 21*
7.	C	*p. 8*	14.	C	*p. 14*			

MATCHING

pp. 9–10

21.	C	22.	D	23.	E	24.	A	25.	B

pp. 12–13

26.	S	27.	P	28.	R	29.	Q	30.	P
31.	O	32.	R	33.	T	34.	Q	35.	O

SHORT ANSWER

p. 5

36. The differential field diagnosis is a listing of the possible primary problems that could cause the chief complaint. The final field diagnosis is the most likely primary problem responsible for the patient's chief complaint, history, and signs and symptoms based upon the patient assessment.

SPECIAL PROJECT: History of the Present Illness

- **O.** (onset of the problem) rapid onset while jogging
- **P.** (provocative/palliative factors) mild pain while deep breathing
- **Q.** (quality of pain) sharp, stabbing
- **R.** (radiation/region of pain) just left of sternum at 3rd intercostal space, with no radiation
- **S.** (severity) 8 on a scale of 1-to-10
- **T.** (time of onset) sudden, with no preceding events
- **AS.** (associated symptoms) none reported
- **PN.** (pertinent negative) denies COPD, asthma, or history of heart problems

CHAPTER 2: Physical Exam Techniques

Section I

CONTENT SELF-EVALUATION

MULTIPLE CHOICE

1.	A	*p. 29*	10.	B	*p. 33*	19.	B	*p. 36*
2.	B	*p. 32*	11.	C	*p. 33*	20.	C	*p. 36*
3.	A	*p. 31*	12.	A	*p. 33*	21.	E	*p. 36*
4.	C	*p. 29*	13.	E	*p. 35*	22.	C	*p. 37*
5.	B	*p. 30*	14.	A	*p. 35*	23.	D	*p. 37*
6.	C	*p. 31*	15.	D	*p. 35*	24.	D	*p. 37*
7.	A	*p. 31*	16.	C	*p. 35*	25.	B	*p. 38*
8.	A	*p. 31*	17.	A	*p. 35*	26.	B	*p. 29*
9.	C	*p. 32*	18.	E	*p. 35*	27.	D	*p. 43*

28.	B	*p. 43*	36.	D	*p. 48*	44.	D	*p. 60*
29.	A	*p. 43*	37.	E	*p. 49*	45.	A	*p. 64*
30.	E	*p. 43*	38.	A	*p. 50*	46.	B	*p. 64*
31.	C	*p. 43*	39.	B	*p. 42*	47.	C	*p. 66*
32.	B	*p. 46*	40.	D	*p. 54*	48.	E	*p. 66*
33.	E	*p. 46*	41.	E	*p. 56*	49.	A	*p. 70*
34.	D	*p. 46*	42.	E	*p. 59*	50.	B	*p. 74*
35.	B	*p. 47*	43.	C	*p. 59*			

SPECIAL PROJECT: Vital Signs

Review pp. 33–37.

Pulse: Evaluate pulse rate, quality (or strength), and rhythm. Pulses should be strong, regular, and have a rate of 60 to 100 per minute in adults.

Respirations: Evaluate rate, effort, and quality (depth and pattern). The respiratory rate should be between 12 to 20 times per minute with minimal effort involved in using the diaphragm and intercostal muscles. Breathing should show a regular rhythm and move about 500 mL with each breath.

Blood pressure: Evaluate the diastolic, systolic, and pulse pressures. The normal systolic blood pressure is 100 to 135, the normal diastolic pressure is 60 to 80, and the pulse pressure is between 30 and 40 mmHg. Blood pressures in premenopausal women are slightly lower.

Temperature: Evaluate the core body temperature. The normal core temperature is about 98.6°F or 37°C.

Section II

MULTIPLE CHOICE

1.	B	*p. 77*	11.	A	*p. 84*	21.	B	*p. 106*
2.	D	*p. 78*	12.	E	*p. 85*	22.	E	*p. 106*
3.	B	*p. 78*	13.	C	*p. 86*	23.	A	*p. 110*
4.	E	*p. 79*	14.	A	*p. 86*	24.	C	*p. 116*
5.	B	*p. 79*	15.	C	*p. 90*	25.	D	*p. 118*
6.	A	*p. 79*	16.	D	*p. 94*	26.	E	*p. 118*
7.	C	*p. 79*	17.	D	*p. 94*	27.	A	*p. 124*
8.	C	*p. 81*	18.	A	*p. 98*	28.	E	*p. 124*
9.	B	*p. 82*	19.	B	*p. 103*	29.	B	*p. 126*
10.	D	*p. 84*	20.	C	*p. 104*	30.	D	*p. 126*

SPECIAL PROJECT: Range of Motion Exercise

Upper Extremity

Joint	Flexion/Extension	Rotation	Other Motion
Wrist	90/70		(Medial/Lateral) 20/45
Elbow	160/0		(Supination/Pronation) 90/90
Shoulder	180/50	(Internal/External) 90/90	(Abduction/Adduction) 180/75

Lower Extremity

Joint	Flexion/Extension	Rotation	Other Motion
Ankle	(Dorsiflex/Plantar Flex) 20/45		(Inversion/Eversion) 30/20
Knee	135/90		
Hip	120/0	(External/Internal) 40/45	(Abduction) 90

Section III

MULTIPLE CHOICE

1.	C	p. 131	15.	C	p. 145
2.	A	p. 131	16.	D	p. 147
3.	D	p. 133	17.	A	p. 148
4.	E	p. 131	18.	E	p. 148
5.	E	p. 133	19.	D	p. 148
6.	E	p. 134	20.	E	p. 148
7.	A	p. 134	21.	A	p. 149
8.	E	p. 136	22.	B	p. 151
9.	B	p. 136	23.	D	p. 152
10.	C	p. 136	24.	C	p. 151
11.	D	p. 137	25.	C	p. 155
12.	D	p. 137	26.	E	p. 158
13.	B	p. 144	27.	A	p. 159
14.	A	p. 144	28.	B	p. 159

29.	B	p. 159
30.	C	p. 159
31.	C	p. 160
32.	E	p. 160
33.	B	p. 160
34.	A	p. 162
35.	B	p. 162
36.	B	p. 162
37.	A	p. 162
38.	D	p. 163
39.	E	p. 165
40.	A	p. 165

MATCHING

See Table 2-11, p. 145.

41.	I, l, m	
42.	II, b, p	
43.	III, h, w	
44.	IV, c, s	
45.	V, g, x	
46.	VI, d, u	

47.	VII, k, q
48.	VIII, a, v
49.	IX, f, t
50.	X, i, n
51.	XI, e, o
52.	XII, j, r

SPECIAL PROJECT: Auscultation Exercise

CHAPTER 3: Patient Assessment in the Field

Section I

CONTENT SELF-EVALUATION

MULTIPLE CHOICE

1.	A	p. 173	11.	A	p. 179	21.	A	p. 186
2.	E	p. 173	12.	D	p. 183	22.	E	p. 186
3.	E	p. 174	13.	B	p. 183	23.	C	p. 187
4.	B	p. 175	14.	A	p. 183	24.	A	p. 188
5.	A	p. 175	15.	B	p. 183	25.	C	p. 188
6.	C	p. 176	16.	D	p. 183	26.	A	p. 188
7.	A	p. 176	17.	E	p. 184	27.	B	p. 190
8.	E	p. 176	18.	C	p. 185	28.	D	p. 191
9.	E	p. 177	19.	E	p. 185	29.	A	p. 195
10.	C	p. 179	20.	C	p. 186	30.	C	p. 195

LISTING

p. 173

31. Scene size-up
32. Initial assessment
33. Focused history and physical exam
34. Detailed physical exam
35. Ongoing assessment

SPECIAL PROJECT: Scene Size-Up Exercise

Possible scene hazards include the following:

A. traffic, unstable vehicle, spilled gasoline/fire, stream contamination, unstable/slippery surfaces, hazardous chemicals, broken glass/jagged metal, hot surfaces
B. structural collapse, debris, confined spaces, electrical hazards, explosion, body substances
C. fast water, drowning, hypothermia

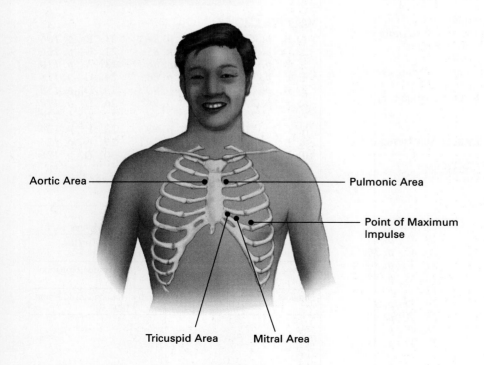

Aortic Area — Pulmonic Area

Point of Maximum Impulse

Tricuspid Area   Mitral Area

Section II

MULTIPLE CHOICE

1.	C	*p. 200*	16.	E	*p. 213*
2.	D	*pp. 200–201*	17.	D	*p. 213*
3.	B	*p. 202*	18.	B	*p. 214*
4.	A	*p. 202*	19.	C	*p. 215*
5.	E	*p. 203*	20.	A	*p. 215*
6.	A	*p. 203*	21.	D	*p. 215*
7.	D	*p. 203*	22.	B	*p. 216*
8.	A	*p. 203*	23.	E	*p. 216*
9.	B	*p. 204*	24.	B	*p. 216*
10.	C	*p. 204*	25.	E	*p. 218*
11.	B	*p. 205*	26.	A	*p. 219*
12.	D	*p. 208*	27.	D	*p. 220*
13.	B	*p. 208*	28.	A	*p. 222*
14.	D	*p. 211*	29.	A	*p. 228*
15.	C	*p. 212*	30.	E	*p. 229*

CHAPTER 4: Clinical Decision Making

CONTENT SELF-EVALUATION

MULTIPLE CHOICE

1.	A	*p. 236*	9.	B	*pp. 238–240*
2.	D	*p. 237*	10.	A	*pp. 239–240*
3.	A	*p. 237*	11.	D	*pp. 242–243*
4.	C	*p. 238*	12.	B	*p. 242*
5.	D	*p. 238*	13.	A	*p. 243*
6.	C	*p. 238*	14.	D	*p. 245*
7.	A	*p. 238*	15.	B	*p. 247*
8.	B	*p. 238*			

MATCHING

pp. 245–246

16.	B	17.	D	18.	A	19.	A	20.	C
21.	B	22.	A	23.	C	24.	A	25.	D

CHAPTER 5: Communications

CONTENT SELF-EVALUATION

MULTIPLE CHOICE

1.	E	*pp. 252–253*	8.	E	*p. 258*	15.	D	*p. 265*
2.	B	*p. 254*	9.	E	*p. 260*	16.	E	*p. 266*
3.	C	*p. 255*	10.	A	*p. 261*	17.	A	*p. 266*
4.	E	*p. 256*	11.	B	*p. 261*	18.	D	*p. 267*
5.	D	*p. 257*	12.	D	*p. 262*	19.	A	*p. 267*
6.	B	*p. 257*	13.	C	*p. 263*	20.	C	*p. 268*
7.	A	*p. 258*	14.	A	*p. 265*			

SPECIAL PROJECT: Documentation: Radio Report/Prehospital Care Report

Your report should include most of the following elements:

Radio message from the scene to medical control:

Unit 89 to Receiving Hospital.

We are at the ball field treating a 13-year-old male who collapsed while playing baseball. He is currently unresponsive to all but painful stimuli, is cool to the touch, and is sweating profusely. Vitals are BP 136/98, pulse 92 and strong, respirations 24 and regular, and pupils equal and slow to react. ECG is showing a normal sinus rhythm. No physical signs of trauma noted, and past medical history is unknown. Oxygen is applied at 12 liters via nonrebreather. Expected ETA, 20 minutes.

Follow-up radio message to Receiving Hospital:

One IV in left forearm is running TKO with NS. Patient now responding to verbal stimuli. Vitals are BP 134/96, pulse 90 and strong, respirations 24. ECG shows normal sinus rhythm. ETA, 10 minutes.

Ambulance run report form:

Please review the accompanying form and check to be sure the form you completed includes the appropriate information. Note that you should include most, if not all, of the information listed on the accompanying sample form. If you have not done this, please review the narrative in the Workbook and determine what is missing from your version. Assure that no important details are left out of the report.

Review the completed form on the following page to ensure that your report includes the appropriate information.

CHAPTER 6: Documentation

CONTENT SELF-EVALUATION

MULTIPLE CHOICE

1.	E	*p. 273*	11.	B	*p. 287*	21.	E	*p. 292*
2.	B	*p. 273*	12.	A	*p. 287*	22.	D	*p. 292*
3.	A	*p. 274*	13.	E	*p. 289*	23.	E	*p. 293*
4.	B	*p. 274*	14.	A	*p. 289*	24.	A	*p. 293*
5.	B	*p. 275*	15.	C	*p. 289*	25.	E	*p. 294*
6.	C	*p. 285*	16.	B	*p. 290*	26.	B	*p. 294*
7.	A	*p. 285*	17.	D	*p. 290*	27.	A	*p. 294*
8.	D	*p. 286*	18.	E	*p. 290*	28.	D	*p. 295*
9.	C	*p. 286*	19.	B	*p. 291*	29.	E	*p. 296*
10.	B	*p. 287*	20.	A	*p. 291*	30.	C	*p. 297*

MATCHING

See pp. 277–294.

31.	P	36.	E	41.	M	46.	V	51.	W
32.	Y	37.	B	42.	J	47.	I	52.	K
33.	L	38.	O	43.	Q	48.	N	53.	S
34.	T	39.	U	44.	G	49.	F	54.	D
35.	A	40.	X	45.	R	50.	C	55.	H

SPECIAL PROJECT: Documentation: Radio Report/Prehospital Care Report

Radio message from the scene to medical control:

Unit 21 to Medical Control. We are attending a male victim of a one-car crash. He was initially unconscious but is now conscious, alert, and oriented. He has a small contusion on his forehead and a small welt on his neck. He was stung by a bee and has had a previous allergic reaction. Vitals are BP 110/76, pulse 90 and strong, respirations 30, and O_2 saturation of 94 percent. There are audible wheezes, and he is complaining of "a lump in the throat." He is on 12 L of O_2 via nonrebreather and has one IV of LR running TKO. A cervical collar has been applied and spinal immobilization is underway.

Follow-up radio message to Community Hospital:

0.3 mg epinephrine SQ and 50 mg Benadryl IM have been administered. Current vitals are BP 122/78, pulse 68 and strong, respirations 22 and regular, O_2 saturation 98 percent. Breath sounds are now clear. ETA is 10 minutes.

Date **Today's Date**	Emergency Medical Services Run Report	Run # **911**

Patient Information	Service Information	Times

Name: **Thompson, Jim**	Agency: **Unit 89**	Rcvd	**15:15**
Address: **Unknown**	Location: **Ballfield**	Enrt	**15:16**
City: St: Zip:	Call Origin: **Dispatch**	Scne	**15:22**
Age: **13** Birth: / / Sex: [**M**][F]	Type: Emrg[**X**] Non[ ] Trnsfr[ ]	LvSn	**15:38**
Nature of Call: **Unconscious person**		ArHsp	**15:57**
Chief Complaint: **Unconsciousness—possible heat exhaustion**		InSv	**16:15**

Description of Current Problem:

The patient collapsed while playing baseball on a very hot, sunny

day. Pt. was found to be cool & diaphoretic, unresponsive to

verbal stimuli, and responsive to painful stimuli. Pupils were

normal in size but slow to react. Physical assessment reveals no

apparent signs of trauma or other medical problem.

Medical Problems

Past		Present
[ ]	Cardiac	[ ]
[ ]	Stroke	[ ]
[ ]	Acute Abdomen	[ ]
[ ]	Diabetes	[ ]
[ ]	Psychiatric	[ ]
[ ]	Epilepsy	[ ]
[ ]	Drug/Alcohol	[ ]
[ ]	Poisoning	[ ]
[ ]	Allergy/Asthma	[ ]
[ ]	Syncope	[ ]
[ ]	Obstetrical	[ ]
[ ]	GYN	[ ]

Other: **Unknown**

Trauma Scr: **n/a**   Glasgow: **6**

On Scene Care: **provided oxygen, removed patient from sun and heat. Attempted IV in right forearm (unsuccessful) started IV in left forearm w/ 16 ga NS – TKO**

First Aid: **pillow was placed under head**

By Whom? **bystanders**

O2 @ **12** L **15:27** Via **NRB**	C-Collar **n/a** :	S-Immob. **n/a**	Stretcher **15:37**

Allergies/Meds: **Unknown**

Past Med Hx: **Unknown**

Time	Pulse	Resp.	BP S/D	LOC	ECG
15:27	R: **92** [**X**][i]	R: **24** [s][l]	**136**/**98**	[a][v][**X**][u]	**Normal Sinus Rhythm**

Care/Comments: **Pt. unresponsive to all but painful stimuli**

15:37	R: **90** [**X**][i]	R: **24** [s][l]	**134**/**96**	[a][**X**][p][u]	**Normal Sinus Rhythm**

Care/Comments: **Pt. became responsive to verbal stimuli**

15:45	R: **88** [**X**][i]	R: **24** [s][l]	**132**/**90**	[**X**][v][p][u]	**Normal Sinus Rhythm**

Care/Comments: **Pt. became fully concious, alert, and oriented**

:	R: [r][i]	R: [s][l]	/	[a][v][p][u]	

Care/Comments:

Destination: **Receiving Hospital**	Personnel:	Certification
Reason:[ ]pt [**X**]Closest [ ]M.D. [ ]Other	1. **Your Name**	[**X**][E][O]
Contacted: [**X**]Radio [ ]Tele [ ]Direct	2. **Steve Phillips**	[P][**X**][O]
Ar Status: [**X**]Better [ ]UnC [ ]Worse	3. **n/a**	[P][E][O]

Ambulance run report:

Please review the accompanying form and check to be sure the form you completed includes the appropriate information. Note that you should include most, if not all, of the information listed on the accompanying sample form. If you have not done this, please review the narrative in the Workbook and determine what is missing from your version. Assure that no important details are left out of the report.

Review the completed form on the following page to ensure that your report includes the appropriate information.

PATIENT ASSESSMENT: Content Review

CONTENT SELF-EVALUATION

CHAPTER 1: THE HISTORY

1. C	p. 5	6. A	p. 9	11. E	p. 15
2. E	p. 6	7. D	p. 10	12. C	p. 16
3. B	p. 7	8. B	p. 11	13. B	p. 18
4. E	p. 8	9. E	p. 13	14. D	p. 21
5. A	p. 8	10. A	p. 15	15. B	p. 24

CHAPTER 2: PHYSICAL EXAM TECHNIQUES

16. D	p. 31	53. B	p. 106	73. E	p. 152
17. D	p. 31	54. A	p. 110	74. A	p. 158
18. B	p. 30	55. B	p. 116	75. B	p. 159
19. B	p. 31	56. E	p. 124	76. C	p. 159
20. B	p. 31	57. D	p. 124	77. D	p. 160
21. C	p. 33	58. A	p. 126	78. A	p. 162
22. B	p. 35	59. D	p. 131	79. D	p. 162
23. B	p. 35	60. C	p. 131	80. D	p. 162
24. B	p. 36	61. E	p. 134	81. C	p. 162
25. C	p. 36	62. C	p. 133	82. B	p. 163
26. C	p. 35	63. A	p. 136	83. A	p. 165
27. D	p. 35	64. C	p. 135	84. B	p. 165
28. E	p. 36	65. C	p. 137		
29. A	p. 37	66. C	p. 145		
30. B	p. 43	67. D	p. 137		
31. E	p. 43	68. A	p. 145		
32. A	p. 43	69. D	p. 145		
33. C	p. 46	70. C	p. 145		
34. E	p. 46	71. A	p. 151		
35. B	p. 50	72. A	p. 149		
36. A	p. 50				
37. C	p. 54				
38. B	p. 66				
39. B	p. 60				
40. B	p. 65				
41. D	p. 70				
42. A	p. 77				
43. D	p. 78				
44. D	p. 79				
45. A	p. 79				
46. D	p. 81				
47. D	p. 85				
48. D	p. 86				
49. E	p. 90				
50. A	p. 94				
51. E	p. 103				
52. E	p. 104				

CHAPTER 3: PATIENT ASSESSMENT IN THE FIELD

85. B	p. 173	95. B	p. 188	105. A	p. 211
86. B	p. 173	96. A	p. 189	106. B	p. 213
87. D	p. 175	97. A	p. 195	107. E	p. 213
88. D	p. 176	98. C	p. 200	108. C	p. 214
89. C	p. 183	99. B	p. 201	109. D	p. 215
90. C	p. 183	100. A	p. 202	110. C	p. 215
91. B	p. 186	101. E	p. 202	111. C	p. 219
92. D	p. 186	102. D	p. 203	112. C	p. 220
93. A	p. 187	103. E	p. 204	113. B	p. 222
94. D	p. 188	104. B	p. 205		

CHAPTER 4: CLINICAL DECISION MAKING

114. B	p. 236	117. E	p. 240	120. D	p. 243
115. C	p. 238	118. A	p. 242	121. B	p. 244
116. A	p. 238	119. C	p. 242		

CHAPTER 5: COMMUNICATIONS

122. E	p. 253	126. B	p. 258	130. C	p. 266
123. C	p. 255	127. A	p. 261	131. D	p. 268
124. D	p. 256	128. C	p. 262		
125. A	p. 257	129. C	p. 266		

CHAPTER 6: DOCUMENTATION

132. D	pp. 272–273	142. C	p. 291
133. C	p. 277	143. E	p. 292
134. C	p. 278	144. A	p. 293
135. D	p. 281	145. C	p. 294
136. B	p. 286	146. D	p. 294
137. B	p. 286	147. C	p. 294
138. D	p. 289	148. E	p. 296
139. C	p. 289	149. C	p. 297
140. A	p. 289	150. E	p. 298
141. B	p. 290		

LOCATING AUSCULTATION POINTS

See p. 84.

Lung Sounds: every 5 cm along the mid-clavicular line
PMI: 5th intercostal space, left mid-clavicular line
S1: lower left sternal border
S2: 2nd intercostal space, near sternum

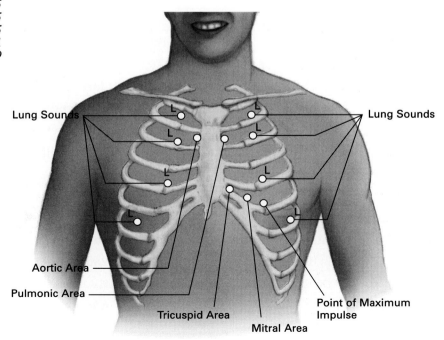

Lung Sounds
Lung Sounds
Aortic Area
Pulmonic Area
Tricuspid Area
Mitral Area
Point of Maximum Impulse

Date **Today's Date**	Emergency Medical Services Run Report	Run # **912**

Patient Information	Service Information		Times	

Name: **William Sobeski**	Agency: **Medic Rescue Unit 21**	Rcvd	**18:32**
Address: **2145 E. Brookline Drive**	Location: **Wildwood & Elm**	Enrt	**18:32**
City: **Rochester** St: Zip:	Call Origin: **Dispatch**	Scne	**18:45**
Age: **28** Birth: / / Sex: [**M**][F]	Type: Emrg[**X**] Non[ ] Trnsfr[ ]	LvSn	**19:02**
Nature of Call: **One-car auto accident**		ArHsp	**19:25**
Chief Complaint: **Head injury—allergic reaction/bee sting**		InSv	**19:55**

Description of Current Problem:

Pt. was apparently stung by a bee, then struck a tree with his auto.

Found unconscious, then awoke. Contusion on his forehead where

it hit the windshield and a small welt on his neck. Pt. complains

of a lump in his throat and mild dyspnea. Mild wheezes on

auscultation. Pt. reports previous life-threatening allergic reaction,

has a prescribed kit but it is at home. Assessment otherwise

unremarkable.

Medical Problems

Past		Present
[ ]	Cardiac	[ ]
[ ]	Stroke	[ ]
[ ]	Acute Abdomen	[ ]
[ ]	Diabetes	[ ]
[ ]	Psychiatric	[ ]
[ ]	Epilepsy	[ ]
[ ]	Drug/Alcohol	[ ]
[ ]	Poisoning	[ ]
[**X**]	Allergy/Asthma	[**X**]
[ ]	Syncope	[ ]
[ ]	Obstetrical	[ ]
[ ]	GYN	[ ]

Other:

Trauma Scr: **16**   Glasgow: **15**

On Scene Care: **0₂, C-Collar, Spinal Imm.**	First Aid: **None**
IV – TKO LR w/ 16 ga R forearm	
0.3 mg Epi SQ, 50 mg Benadryl IM	
	By Whom?

02 @ **12** L **18:52** Via **NRB**	C-Collar **18:50**	S-Immob. **18:52**	Stretcher **18:55**

Allergies/Meds: **Bee sting, no other allergies known**	Past Med Hx: **Bee sting and reaction 2 yrs ago no other history noted.**

Time	Pulse		Resp.		BP S/D	LOC	ECG
18:52	R: **90**	[**X**][i]	R: **30**	[s][l]	**110/76**	[**X**][v][p][u]	**Normal Sinus Rhythm**

Care/Comments: **IV initiated via protocol – 16 ga R forearm, audible wheezes, SaO₂ 94%**

18:59	R: **78**	[**X**][i]	R: **24**	[s][l]	**118/88**	[**X**][v][p][u]	**Normal Sinus Rhythm**

Care/Comments: **Epi & Benadryl administered, SaO₂ 99%, wheezes gone**

19:02	R: **68**	[**X**][i]	R: **22**	[s][l]	**122/78**	[**X**][v][p][u]	**Normal Sinus Rhythm**

Care/Comments: **SaO₂ 98%**

19:20	R: **86**	[**X**][i]	R: **24**	[s][l]	**122/80**	[**X**][v][p][u]	**Normal Sinus Rhythm**

Care/Comments: **Wheezes reduced, SaO₂ 98%**

Destination: **Community Hospital**	Personnel:	Certification
Reason:[**X**]pt [ ]Closest [ ]M.D. [ ]Other	1. **Your Name**	[**R**][E][O]
Contacted: [**X**]Radio [ ]Tele [ ]Direct	2. **Mike Grailing**	[**R**][E][O]
Ar Status: [**X**]Better [ ]UnC [ ]Worse	3. **n/a**	[P][E][O]

Fill in the Blanks
See pp. 277–284.

1. chief complaint
2. history of present illness
3. shortness of breath
4. atherosclerotic heart disease
5. hepatitis B virus
6. paroxysmal nocturnal dyspnea
7. nitroglycerine
8. posterior axillary line
9. complete blood count
10. point of maximal impulse
11. alert and oriented
12. pack/years
13. within normal limits
14. bag-valve mask
15. endotracheal tube
16. nothing by mouth
17. treatment
18. keep vein open
19. subcutaneous
20. bundle branch block

CROSSWORD PUZZLE

Across / Down answers as filled in the grid:

- 2 Across: TACHYCARDIA
- 5 Across: LESION
- 8 Across: WHEEZES
- 9 Across: CARDIAC
- 11 Across: CHIEF
- 14 Across: ASCITES
- 15 Across: LIBEL
- 16 Across: HEPA
- 18 Across: REFLEX
- 19 Across: DELIRIUM
- 20 Across: STRIDOR
- 21 Across: HEENT
- 22 Across: ALS

Down answers (reading the letters in the grid):

- 1: E
- TIDAL, HO, RAU, BUIO, CUOEL, COLUM, CRS I, MMS, FILD, ACUITY

National Registry of Emergency Medical Technicians

PRACTICAL EVALUATION FORMS

The forms on the next pages are provided to help you identify common criteria by which you will be evaluated. It may be valuable to review your practical skills by using these sheets during your class practice sessions and as you review those skills before class, state, and any national testing. Evaluation forms will often vary: however, many of the important elements of paramedic practice are common to all forms.

EMT-PARAMEDIC FORMS

The following skill instruments for the EMT-Paramedic level were developed by the National Registry of EMTs. They are in draft format and have not yet been approved for use in Advanced Level National Registry examinations.

EMT-BASIC FORMS

The skill instruments for the EMT-Basic level reproduced on the following pages have been approved by the National Registry of EMTs.

The author wishes to thank the National Registry for the use of these forms and for their continuing efforts to improve the quality of prehospital emergency medical care.

EMT-Paramedic Form

National Registry of Emergency Medical Technicians
Advanced Level Practical Examinations

PATIENT ASSESSMENT—TRAUMA

Note: Areas denoted by ** may be integrated within sequence of Initial Assessment	Possible Points	Points Awarded
Takes or verbalizes body substance isolation precautions	1	
SCENE SIZE-UP		
Determines the scene/situation is safe	1	
Determines the mechanism of injury/nature of illness	1	
Determines the number of patients	1	
Requests additional help if necessary	1	
Considers stabilization of spine	1	
INITIAL ASSESSMENT/RESUSCITATION		
Verbalizes general impression of patient	1	
Determines responsiveness/level of consciousness	1	
Determines chief complaint/apparent life-threats	1	
Airway —Opens and assesses airway (1 point)　　—Inserts adjunct as indicated (1 point)	2	
Breathing —Assess breathing (1 point) —Assures adequate ventilation (1 point) —Initiates appropriate oxygen therapy (1 point) —Manages any injury which may compromise breathing/ventilation (1 point)	4	
Circulation —Checks pulse (1 point) —Assess skin (either skin color, temperature or condition) (1 point) —Assesses for and controls major bleeding if present (1 point) —Initiates shock management (1 point)	4	
Identifies priority patients/makes transport decision	1	
FOCUSED HISTORY AND PHYSICAL EXAMINATION / RAPID TRAUMA ASSESSMENT		
Selects appropriate assessment	1	
Obtains, or directs assistant to obtain, baseline vital signs	1	
Obtains SAMPLE history	1	
DETAILED PHYSICAL EXAMINATION		
Head —Inspects mouth**, nose**, and assesses facial area (1 point) —Inspects and palpates scalp and ears (1 point) —Assesses eyes for PEARRL** (1 point)	3	
Neck** —Checks position of trachea (1 point) —Checks jugular veins (1 point) —Palpates cervical spine (1 point)	3	
Chest** —Inspects chest (1 point) —Palpates chest (1 point) —Auscultates chest (1 point)	3	
Abdomen/pelvis** —Inspects and palpates abdomen (1 point) —Assesses pelvis (1 point) —Verbalizes assessment of genitalia/perineum as needed (1 point)	3	
Lower extremities** —Inspects, palpates, and assesses motor, sensory, and circulatory functions (1 point/leg)	2	
Upper extremities** —Inspects, palpates, and assesses motor, sensory, and circulatory functions (1 point/arm)	2	
Posterior thorax, lumbar, and buttocks** —Inspects and palpates posterior thorax (1 point) —Inspects and palpates lumbar and buttocks area (1 point)	2	
Manages secondary injuries and wounds appropriately (1 point/injury or wound)	1	
Ongoing assessment (1 point)	1	
TOTAL	43	

CRITICAL CRITERIA

____ Failure to initiate or call for transport of the patient within 10 minute time limit

____ Failure to take or verbalize body substance isolation precautions

____ Failure to determine scene safety

____ Failure to assess for and provide spinal protection when indicated

____ Failure to voice and ultimately provide high concentration of oxygen

____ Failure to find or appropriately manage problems associated with airway, breathing, hemorrhage, or shock (hypoperfusion)

____ Failure to differentiate patient's need for immediate transportation versus continued assessment and treatment at the scene

____ Does other detailed or focused history or physical examination before assessing and treating threats to airway, breathing, and circulation

____ Orders a dangerous or inappropriate intervention

EMT-Paramedic Form

National Registry of Emergency Medical Technicians
Advanced Level Practical Examinations

PATIENT ASSESSMENT—MEDICAL

	Possible Points	Points Awarded
Takes or verbalizes body substance isolation precautions	1	
SCENE SIZE-UP		
Determines the scene/situation is safe	1	
Determines the mechanism of injury/nature of illness	1	
Determines the number of patients	1	
Requests additional help if necessary	1	
Considers stabilization of spine	1	
INITIAL ASSESSMENT		
Verbalizes general impression of patient	1	
Determines responsiveness/level of consciousness	1	
Determines chief complaint/apparent life-threats	1	
Assesses airway and breathing —Assessment (1 point) —Assures adequate ventilation of patient (1 point) —Initiates appropriate oxygen therapy (1 point)	3	
Assesses circulation —Assesses/controls major bleeding (1 point) —Assesses skin (either skin color, temperature or condition) (1 point) —Assesses pulse (1 point)	3	
Identifies priority patients/makes transport decision	1	
FOCUSED HISTORY AND PHYSICAL EXAMINATION / RAPID ASSESSMENT		
History of present illness —Onset (1 point) —Severity (1 point) —Provocation (1 point) —Time (1 point) —Quality (1 point) —Clarify questions (2 points) —Radiation (1 point)	8	
Past medical history —Allergies (1 point) —Last oral intake (1 point) —Medications (1 point) —Events leading to present illness (1 point) —Past pertinent history (1 point)	5	
Performs focused physical examination (assess affected body part/system or, if indicated, completes rapid assessment) —Cardiovascular —Integumentary —Pulmonary —GI/GU —Neurological —Reproductive —Musculoskeletal —Psychological/Social	5	
Vital signs —Pulse (1 point) —Respiratory rate & quality (1 point each) —Blood pressure (1 point) —AVPU (1 point)	5	
Diagnostics	2	
States field impression of patient	1	
Verbalizes treatment plan for patient and calls for appropriate intervention(s)	1	
Transport decision re-evaluated	1	
ONGOING ASSESSMENT		
Repeats initial assessment	1	
Repeats vital signs	1	
Evaluates response to treatments	1	
Repeats focused assessment regarding patient complaint or injuries	1	
TOTAL	48	

CRITICAL CRITERIA

___ Failure to take or verbalize body substance isolation precautions
___ Failure to determine scene safety
___ Failure to voice and ultimately provide appropriate oxygen therapy
___ Failure to find or appropriately manage problems associated with airway, breathing, hemorrhage, or shock (hypoperfusion)
___ Failure to differentiate patient's need for immediate transportation versus continued assessment and treatment at the scene
___ Does other detailed or focused history or physical examination before assessing and treating threats to airway, breathing, and circulation
___ Failure to determine the patient's primary problem
___ Orders a dangerous or inappropriate intervention

EMT-Basic Form

PATIENT ASSESSMENT/MANAGEMENT—TRAUMA

Start Time:_____
Stop Time:_____ Date:_____
Candidate's Name:_____
Evaluator's Name:_____

		Points Possible	Points Awarded
Takes, or verbalizes, body substance isolation precautions		1	
SCENE SIZE-UP			
Determines the scene is safe		1	
Determines the mechanism of injury		1	
Determines the number of patients		1	
Requests additional help if necessary		1	
Considers stabilization of spine		1	
INITIAL ASSESSMENT			
Verbalizes general impression of patient		1	
Determines responsiveness/level of consciousness		1	
Determines chief complaint/apparent life threats		1	
Assesses airway and breathing	Assessment	1	
	Initiates appropriate oxygen therapy	1	
	Assures adequate ventilation	1	
	Injury management	1	
Assesses circulation	Assesses/controls major bleeding	1	
	Assesses pulse	1	
	Assesses skin (color, temperature, and condition)	1	
Identifies priority patients/makes transport decision		1	
FOCUSED HISTORY AND PHYSICAL EXAM/RAPID TRAUMA ASSESSMENT			
Selects appropriate assessment (**focused or rapid assessment**)		1	
Obtains or directs assistant to obtain baseline vital signs		1	
Obtains S.A.M.P.L.E. history		1	
DETAILED PHYSICAL EXAMINATION			
Assesses the head	Inspects and palpates the scalp and ears	1	
	Assesses the eyes	1	
	Assesses the facial areas including oral and nasal areas	1	
Assesses the neck	Inspects and palpates the neck	1	
	Assesses for JVD	1	
	Assesses for tracheal deviation	1	
Assesses the chest	Inspects	1	
	Palpates	1	
	Auscultates	1	
Assesses the abdomen/pelvis	Assesses the abdomen	1	
	Assesses the pelvis	1	
	Verbalizes assessment of genitalia/perineum as needed	1	
Assesses the extremities	1 point for each extremity includes inspection, palpation, and assessment of motor, sensory and circulatory function	4	
Assesses the posterior	Assesses thorax	1	
	Assesses lumbar	1	
Manages secondary injuries and wounds appropriately **1 point for appropriate management of secondary injury/wound**		1	
Verbalizes re-assessment of the vital signs		1	
	Total:	40	

Critical Criteria

___ Did not take, or verbalize, body substance isolation precautions
___ Did not determine scene safety.
___ Did not assess for spinal protection
___ Did not provide for spinal protection when indicated
___ Did not provide high concentration of oxygen
___ Did not find, or manage, problems associated with airway, breathing, hemorrhage or shock (hypoperfusion)
___ Did not differentiate patient's need for transportation versus continued assessment at the scene
___ Did other detailed physical examination before assessing airway, breathing, and circulation
___ Did not transport patient within (10) minute time limit

EMT-Basic Form

PATIENT ASSESSMENT/MANAGEMENT—MEDICAL

Start Time:_____
Stop Time:_____   Date:_____
Candidate's Name:_____
Evaluator's Name:_____

	Points Possible	Points Awarded
Takes, or verbalizes, body substance isolation precautions	1	
SCENE SIZE-UP		
Determines the scene is safe	1	
Determines the mechanism of injury/nature of illness	1	
Determines the number of patients	1	
Requests additional help if necessary	1	
Considers stabilization of spine	1	
INITIAL ASSESSMENT		
Verbalizes general impression of patient	1	
Determines responsiveness/level of consciousness	1	
Determines chief complaint/apparent life threats	1	
Assesses airway and breathing — Assessment	1	
Initiates appropriate oxygen therapy	1	
Assures adequate ventilation	1	
Assesses circulation — Assesses/controls major bleeding	1	
Assesses pulse	1	
Assesses skin (color, temperature, and condition)	1	
Identifies priority patients/makes transport decision	1	
FOCUSED HISTORY AND PHYSICAL EXAM/RAPID ASSESSMENT		
Signs and symptoms (*Assesses history of present illness*)	1	

Respiratory	Cardiac	Altered Mental Status	Allergic Reaction	Poisoning/ Overdose	Environmental Emergency	Obstetrics	Behavioral
•Onset? •Provokes? •Quality? •Radiates? •Severity? •Time? •Interventions?	•Onset? •Provokes? •Quality? •Radiates? •Severity? •Time? •Interventions?	•Description of the episode •Onset? •Duration? •Associated symptoms? •Evidence of trauma? •Interventions? •Seizures? •Fever?	•History of allergies? •What were you exposed to? •How were you exposed? •Effects? •Progression? •Interventions?	•Substance? •When did you ingest/become exposed? •How much did you ingest? •Over what time period? •Interventions? •Estimated weight?	•Source? •Environment? •Duration? •Loss of consciousness? •Effects— General or local?	•Are you pregnant? •How long have you been pregnant? •Pain or contractions? •Bleeding or discharge? •Do you feel the need to push? •Last menstrual period?	•How do you feel? •Determine suicidal tendencies •Is the patient a threat to self or others? •Is there a medical problem? •Interventions?

	Points Possible	Points Awarded
Allergies		
Medications	1	
Past pertinent history	1	
Last oral intake	1	
Events leading to present illness (rule out trauma)	1	
Performs focused physical examination (*assesses affected body part/system or, if indicated, completes rapid assessment*)	1	
Vitals (obtains baseline vital signs)	1	
Interventions (*obtains medical direction or verbalizes standing order for medication interventions and verbalizes proper additional intervention/treatment*)	1	
Transport (re-evaluates transport decision)	1	
Verbalizes the consideration for completing a detailed physical examination	1	
ONGOING ASSESSMENT (verbalized)		
Repeats initial assessment	1	
Repeats vital signs	1	
Repeats focused assessment regarding patient complaint or injuries	1	
Total:	30	

Critical Criteria

___ Did not take, or verbalize, body substance isolation precautions when necessary
___ Did not determine scene safety
___ Did not obtain medical direction or verbalize standing orders for medication interventions
___ Did not provide high concentration of oxygen
___ Did not find or manage problems associated with airway, breathing, hemorrhage or shock (hypoperfusion)
___ Did not differentiate patient's need for transportation versus continued assessment at the scene
___ Did detailed or focused history/physical examination before assessing airway, breathing and circulation
___ Did not ask questions about the present illness
___ Administered a dangerous or inappropriate intervention

Paramedic Care: Principles & Practice

PATIENT ASSESSMENT

Comment Form

In the space below, please provide any suggestions or comments regarding either the Paramedic Care Patient Assessment *textbook or the accompanying workbook. Please enter your phone number in case we have any questions.*

Name: _____   Phone: _____ - _____ - _____

Text [   ] or Workbook [   ]   Page number _____

_____
_____
_____
_____
_____

Text [   ] or Workbook [   ]   Page number _____

_____
_____
_____
_____
_____

Text [   ] or Workbook [   ]   Page number _____

_____
_____
_____
_____
_____

Text [   ] or Workbook [   ]   Page number _____

_____
_____
_____
_____
_____

Please fold this form in thirds and tape it closed. Place your return address on the form and apply the appropriate postage.

Thank you for your input.   Robert S. Porter   Bryan E. Bledsoe   Richard A. Cherry fold ....

_____

_____   Stamp

_____

PARAMEDIC CARE: PRINCIPLES & PRACTICE
BRADY/PRENTICE HALL HEALTH
MARKETING DEPARTMENT
ONE LAKE STREET
UPPER SADDLE RIVER, NJ   07458

fold ....

PATIENT SCENARIO FLASH CARDS

In order to help you learn the process of investigating the chief complaint and obtaining the past medical history, we have included a series of flash cards. Each one contains the dispatch and scene size-up information and then asks you to question either the patient's chief complaint or the past medical history.

Using the flash cards is a two-person exercise. Work with another member of your class, a paramedic or EMT from your service, or with someone else knowledgeable in emergency medical care. Cut the cards and shuffle them. Have your partner choose a card at random and read the dispatch and scene survey information aloud to you. He or she should read the patient information to him- or herself and prepare to play the role of the patient. You should then try to determine the patient history by questioning him or her using the elements of the SAMPLE mnemonic. Your partner should then choose other cards and the two of you repeat the exercise until you feel comfortable in gathering the patient history.

Then have your partner repeat the exercise, reading the dispatch and scene survey information and role playing the part of the patient with symptoms associated with the chief complaint. You should then question him or her about the chief complaint using the OPQRST-ASPN mnemonic. When you feel comfortable with the process of questioning for the chief complaint, repeat the exercise with your partner using information on both sides of the card. When you have gathered all the information you can, create a patient report like the one you would provide when arriving at the emergency department with your patient. Also attempt to determine the field diagnosis for the patient (listed at the bottom of the chief complaint card). Repeat the exercise until you are comfortable with the entire process.

PATIENT HISTORY

The patient history examines critical elements of the patient's past medical history, including the elements of the SAMPLE history mnemonic. (The S, for signs and symptoms, is investigated during the questioning about the chief complaint.)

A—allergies	Ask about any allergies or adverse reactions to drugs, foods, etc.
M—medications	Ask about any prescribed medications, then over-the-counter ones.
P—past medical history	Ask about recent surgeries, hospitalizations, and physician care.
L—last oral intake	Ask about the most recent meal and any fluids ingested.
E—events before the incident	Ask about activities and symptoms preceding the incident.

CHIEF COMPLAINT

During the investigation of the chief complaint, question the patient about the major symptoms of the problem to help form a field diagnosis. Investigate your patient's complaints by using the OPQRST-ASPN mnemonic.

O (onset)	Ask about how the symptoms developed and what the patient was doing at the time.
P (palliation/provocation)	Ask about what makes the symptoms better or worse.
Q (quality)	Ask the patient to describe the nature of the pain or discomfort.
R (region/radiation)	Ask where the symptom and related symptoms are found.
S (severity)	Ask the patient to rate the pain on a scale from 1 to 10 (worst pain).
T (time)	Ask about when the symptoms first appeared and how they progressed.
AS (associated symptoms)	Ask about other or associated symptoms.
PN (pertinent negatives)	Investigate likely and related signs and symptoms.

During this exercise, do not try to develop standard questions for each element of the investigation. Rather, let your patient's condition, the nature of the problem, and—later during your career—your experience guide your questioning to garner the pertinent medical information.

CARD 1 PATIENT HISTORY

Dispatch Information: Responding to a residence for a patient complaining of chest pain.

Scene Survey: Small but clean home with the patient seated on the couch, in obvious pain, and clenching his chest; no hazards noted.

Medical History
A—anesthetic at the dentist's office ("caine" family)
M—nitroglycerine and calcium supplements
P—sees his doctor yearly but doesn't have any medical problems
L—breakfast an hour ago, 2 eggs, toast and coffee
E—watching television, nothing unusual

CARD 2 PATIENT HISTORY

Dispatch Information: Responding to a local movie theater for a man with abdominal pain.

Scene Survey: A crowd surrounds a man seated in the lobby; no hazards noted.

Medical History
A—doesn't know of any
M—none
P—pelvic fracture 3 years ago (auto accident)
L—a large prime rib dinner 2 hours ago with a couple of gin and tonics
E—just sitting in the movie when this pain began and became progressively worse

CARD 3 PATIENT HISTORY

Dispatch Information: Seizure at the penny arcade.

Scene Survey: You are directed to the manager's office where you find a rather lethargic young female; no hazards are noted.

Medical History
A—she doesn't know
M—Dilantin® and phenobarbital, but hasn't been taking them
P—serious auto accident and then seizures
L—had a light lunch an hour ago
E—just felt warm, then blacked out

CARD 1 CHIEF COMPLAINT

Chief Complaint
O—sudden onset, 15 minutes ago
P—nothing, including nitro, makes it better or worse
Q—dull
R—substernal with some right arm numbness
S—12 out of 10, more than ever before
T—while watching TV
AS—some nausea
PN—no dizziness or dyspnea

(Field Diagnosis: Myocardial infarction)

CARD 2 CHIEF COMPLAINT

Chief Complaint
O—gradual onset; started about 1 hour ago and got worse
P—bending over gives some relief
Q—dull, cramping-like pain
R—right upper quadrant with some pain in the right shoulder
S—10 on a scale of 1 to 10
T—ate a prime rib dinner 2 hours ago, watching a movie
AS—some nausea
PN—none noted

(Field Diagnosis: Gallbladder inflammation [*Cholecycstitis*])

CARD 3 CHIEF COMPLAINT

Chief Complaint
O—just had a warm feeling, then blacked out
P—none
Q—bystander states the patient tensed, arched her back, then seized
R—bystander states seizure began with everything shaking
S—generalized motor seizure
T—watching the lights on an arcade game, then experienced a warm feeling, collapsed, and awoke feeling tired
AS—tongue bitten and bleeding
PN—no headache

(Field Diagnosis: Epilepsy)

CARD 4 PATIENT HISTORY

Dispatch Information: Responding to a resident at a nursing home with problems breathing.

Scene Survey: You are directed by staff to an elderly patient, in bed on oxygen, and in noticeable distress; no hazards noted.

Medical History
A—shellfish
M—28% oxygen via Venturi mask
P—emphysema (30 pack/year smoker) and a weak heart
L—light breakfast 4 hours ago and a glass of milk an hour ago
E—just lying here, knitting

CARD 5 PATIENT HISTORY

Dispatch Information: Patient with abdominal pain at the high school.

Scene Survey: At the high school nurse's office, you find a young female teenager curled up on the couch; no hazards noted.

Medical History
A—none
M—antibiotic for infection
P—none
L—breakfast this morning
E—twinge of pain began earlier this morning and grew worse

CARD 6 PATIENT HISTORY

Dispatch Information: Dispatched to the local library for a man who has collapsed.

Scene Survey
An older, well-dressed gentleman is lying on the floor in a pool of his own urine; no hazards noted.

Medical History
A—none known
M—daily aspirin and digitalis for heart disease
P—cardiac dysrhythmias
L—dinner about an hour ago
E—just sitting and reading when a headache developed

CARD 4 CHIEF COMPLAINT

Chief Complaint
O—slow progression of difficulty breathing
P—any movement or stress makes it worse
Q—general fatigue and a "tight" chest
R—limited to the chest
S—intensity of dyspnea, 8 out of 10
T—progressed slowly, started two hours ago
AS—none
PN—no pitting edema or jugular vein distension

(Field Diagnosis: Exacerbation of COPD)

CARD 5 CHIEF COMPLAINT

Chief Complaint
O—the pain began this morning and has gradually increased
P—somewhat more comfortable in the fetal position
Q—"crampy"
R—localized to the left lower quadrant
S—pain is 9 on a scale of 1-to-10
T—gradually increasing since morning, nothing unusual in diet or activity
AS—last period spotty, not the usual flow
PN—appendix was removed last year

(Field Diagnosis: Ectopic pregnancy)

CARD 6 CHIEF COMPLAINT

Chief Complaint
O—developed a headache, and then just collapsed
P—nothing affects the pain or paralysis
Q—throbbing headache, full one-sided paralysis
R—left-sided paralysis of both extremities
S—headache pain is 10 on a 1-to-10 scale
T—reading preceded symptoms
AS—incontinence, difficulty speaking and understanding
PN—pupils normal and reactive

(Field Diagnosis: CVA—stroke)

Card 7 Patient History

Dispatch Information: Proceed to a local restaurant for an unruly and disoriented person.

Scene Survey: Police are already at the scene where a young woman who looks anxious is seated in a booth; no hazards noted.

Medical History
A—sulfa drugs
M—insulin subcutaneously twice per day
P—juvenile-onset (Type I) diabetes
L—ate a small breakfast about 8 hours ago
E—took insulin just after breakfast

Card 8 Patient History

Dispatch Information: Dispatched to high-school gym for a "weak student."

Scene Survey: A young male is seated on the bleachers in obvious distress; no hazards noted.

Medical History
A—tetanus toxoid
M—none
P—none but had sports physical last month, everything was OK
L—a good-sized lunch about an hour ago
E—sudden chest pain while running in the gym

Card 9 Patient History

Dispatch Information: Dispatched to a residence for a patient with chest pain and dyspnea; time is 0200.

Scene Survey: The patient's wife directs you to the bedroom where a middle-aged male is experiencing dyspnea; no hazards noted.

Medical History
A—eggs and egg products
M—antibiotics
P—hip replacement 3 weeks ago, bed rest
L—dinner, a sandwich, and a glass of milk
E—awakened from sleep by pain and difficulty breathing

CARD 7 CHIEF COMPLAINT

Chief Complaint
O—gradual onset of confusion, then combativeness
P—hard candy has calmed her somewhat
Q—disoriented to time and place
R—not applicable
S—friends say this is the worst they have seen her
T—slow progression of confusion, then combativeness
AS—alcohol-like odor on breath
PN—none

(Field diagnosis: Insulin shock)

CARD 8 CHIEF COMPLAINT

Chief Complaint
O—sudden onset of chest pain
P—deep breathing increases pain
Q—"stabbing"
R—left chest only
S—pain is about 7 on 1-to-10 scale, moderate dyspnea
T—after running took a deep breath, then started
AS—none
PN—no heart history or irregular pulse

(Field Diagnosis: Spontaneous pneumothorax)

CARD 9 CHIEF COMPLAINT

Chief Complaint
O—sudden mild chest pain; patient states, "I can't catch my breath"
P—nothing increases or decreases pain or dyspnea
Q—sharp and stabbing
R—left chest area
S—pain is 4 on a 1-to-10 scale
T—while asleep, sudden and nonprogressive
AS—ashen skin
PN—no dull substernal pain, no history of asthma or COPD

(Field Diagnosis: Pulmonary embolism)